before
& after

before
& after

Living and Eating Well
After Weight-Loss Surgery

Second Revised Edition

SUSAN MARIA LEACH

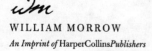
WILLIAM MORROW
An Imprint of HarperCollins*Publishers*

This book is dedicated to my husband, Ty, who loves me for my heart no matter what size I am; and to my mother, Beatrice, who I wish were here to share my happiness. I can now look in the mirror and find her smile in my face.

BEFORE & AFTER (SECOND REVISED EDITION). Copyright © 2004, 2007, 2012 by Susan Maria Leach. All rights reserved. Printed in the United States of America. No part of this book may be used or reproduced in any manner whatsoever without written permission except in the case of brief quotations embodied in critical articles and reviews. For information address HarperCollins Publishers, 10 East 53rd Street, New York, NY 10022.

HarperCollins books may be purchased for educational, business, or sales promotional use. For information please write: Special Markets Department, HarperCollins Publishers, 10 East 53rd Street, New York, NY 10022.

FIRST EDITION

Library of Congress Cataloging-in-Publication Data has been applied for.

ISBN 978-0-06-223999-0

12   13   14   15   16   DIX/RRD   10   9   8   7   6   5   4   3   2   1

contents

acknowledgments

Thank you to Dr. Carlos Carrasquilla for caring enough to perfect this amazing surgery.

Special thanks to:

John, who, I will admit, is as good a cook as I am (except for Key lime pie). I would not have taken a picture of a speedometer while driving at a ridiculously high rate of speed on the Autobahn for anyone but you.

Daddy and Diane, for taste testing all of my sugar-free desserts on Sundays. I love you both.

Jo, for having the guts to make a change. I am so happy for your new life and that you allow me to be a part of it.

Harriet Bell, for recognizing how many people this project will help and for allowing me to keep my own voice. I am lucky to have worked with you.

The entire staff at HarperCollins who have helped me turn a folder full of notes and recipes into my new life and passion.

Tania, who has been there for me from the very beginning; my steadfast and loyal BeforeAndAfterHelp.com message board believers, who volunteer their time and have helped tens of thousands of people find their way; Dana and Lexi; Deb and Liz.

I am also thankful for and appreciative of every person who has worked with us at BE in Florida—you have all given of yourself in order to help others.

foreword

Obesity is a worldwide epidemic, and is rampant in the United States. It is newly recognized as a major disease. Obesity not only affects the individual's physical appearance, but also increases health risks and the incidence of death. To know that in the United States alone, there are more than 300,000 preventable deaths yearly, about 34 each hour, is very serious and frightening.

There is a considerable list of diseases called *comorbidities* associated with obesity, which aggravate an already serious situation. The comorbid complications could be psychological, social, economic, and, of greater concern, medical. The list includes illnesses such as diabetes, hypertension, coronary artery disease, respiratory problems, reflux, and an extended sublist of illnesses with different degrees of seriousness. The gravity of the health status varies with the increase of weight in the individual.

To the patients with a status of "morbid obesity"—100 pounds or more above their ideal weight—the treatment of choice becomes surgery, since nonsurgical methods are projected to have an almost total failure rate. Several procedures have been used for weight control. The most common procedure today is the gastric bypass, considered the gold standard of bariatric surgery.

Historically, we have used different types of surgery to obtain and maintain weight loss. We have created malabsorption, physical restriction of the intake of food, and a combination of these two procedures, with variations developed by individual surgeons.

The results after gastric bypass surgery have been extraordinary, not only with the appearance of the patient, but also with improvement or correction of the health risks. In our center, together with my partners, I have been very happy with the results during the last few years. We have operated on more than 1,800 patients and find that they've lost an average of 71 percent of their excess weight in the first twelve months. Among the patients with type 2 diabetes, 99 percent of them have stopped taking medication and enjoy normal blood sugar levels. Of the hypertensive, 90 percent of patients have returned to normal blood pressure levels, allowing them to discontinue their medications. Other problems such as sleep apnea have also been corrected or improved.

Lately, an international study of the obese population from Sweden, Italy, Australia, and the United States have reported a more than 50 percent decrease in deaths of those obese patients who had bariatric surgery.

Patients such as Susan Leach, who are interested in improving their quality of life both physically and emotionally, come to us for information to help them achieve their goals. Those who meet the criteria for bariatric surgery and make the decision to proceed on this journey are given a road map to guide them through. Should they choose to continue to move forward, they will have a surgical consultation and psychological and medical clearance. Once this has been accomplished they proceed with surgery and are on the road to a healthier, happier, and slimmer life. As they approach each crossroad, the decision as to which road to take ultimately becomes theirs.

In the practice of bariatric surgery, with the establishment of dedicated and specialized centers, the great majority of the patients have an ongoing patient-physician relationship. The patients' relationships to each other are also fascinating; they bond together in a fraternity, exchanging information and assistance. It gives us great pleasure and becomes a source of pride to see the changes in these patients, not only in their obvious physical development but also in their health status and new, self-confident personalities.

With Susan, we have seen her radiance and beauty reflected in the eyes of her admiring husband. Her energetic personality exudes assurance, confidence, and the enthusiasm of someone who wants to share her positive experience with others in her situation. Susan relates the story of her life, and at the same time organizes this book to help other patients in that fraternity to facilitate their further success and happiness. Since Susan has personally made that journey, it was her desire to assist her fellow travelers on their way. Realizing that adaptation to certain dietary requirements may be more difficult for some than others, Susan has written this excellent and much-needed book.

In her diary, Susan tells readers how she handled her range of emotions from her decision to undergo surgery to the panic she felt when taking her first drink of water, to later, when she could enjoy only small portions of decadent meals while traveling. Through her encouragement and her recipes, Susan shows how others can discover the pleasures of cooking and eating while maintaining their dietary limitations.

Susan's book shows people who are used to big, rich, and indulgent meals how to adapt their cooking to include healthier choices without losing flavor or feeling deprived. In *Before & After* Susan teaches the reader how to make the necessary dietary changes from day one post-op. Starting with protein shakes, and moving on to "Soups, Purees, and Other Soft Foods," she progresses to more elaborate meals while at the same time maintaining the crucial nutritional requirements. Other patients can discover and enjoy the pleasure of cooking while maintaining the limitations of the "rules of the game."

At one of our regular support group meetings, Susan delighted the members with samples of her low-carbohydrate desserts. As the desserts disappeared before my eyes, I couldn't help noticing the reactions of the group members, who expressed pleasure and surprise in knowing they can enjoy good food without hindering their progress or compromising their health.

If you are considering obesity surgery, my advice is to find an established, dedicated, specialized center with experienced surgeons who provide adequate follow-up with dietary and psychological support. Insist that the surgeon and the team educate you on all aspects of this disease and treatment. Then, prepare yourself for the lifetime adjustments necessary for successful completion of your goal. Books like this one are an excellent guide and assistance for any prospective patient. There are several factors that contribute to the success following this type of surgery. The expertise and dedication of the surgeon and his/her team, a good pre-operative education and the willingness of the patient to follow the advice are things to keep in mind. By arming yourself with Susan's book, you will find the journey a lot more pleasurable.

—Carlos Carrasquilla, M.D., F.A.C.S., director, Florida
Center for Surgical Weight Control, P.A.

a note from a nutritionist

In the fast-growing area of gastric bypass surgery, new information on the subject is vital. As a dietitian in a bariatric surgeon's office, I have worked with more than 400 gastric bypass patients a year. There is a clear need for more advice on how to prepare appetizing foods post-operatively that will appeal to people. Having this surgery should not and does not mean that once-loved foods can no longer be enjoyed. This book is full of recipes to create meals and treats that are tastier than the foods many people may have had even prior to surgery.

When I reviewed the book and its recipes, I was seeing it from a nutritional perspective. I was very impressed (and a little surprised) by how well the recipes align with the guidelines developed by the American Society of Bariatric Surgery. These recipes are prepared without the addition of sugar, which is restricted in the bypass patient due to the adverse reaction it may cause. Susan Leach is careful with the carbohydrate content of the foods that are prepared. This is important because carbohydrates are restricted in the post–gastric bypass patient; fewer carbs makes room in the small stomach for more protein. Many of her recipes are also high in protein, which is a staple of the post–gastric bypass diet. While this book was written with the gastric bypass patient in mind, it can be used by anyone looking for delicious recipes that promote a healthy weight and lifestyle.

—Jennifer Pereira, R.D., LD/N

preface to the 2012 edition

While I'm very happy with life after weight-loss surgery, I was happy with my life *before* weight-loss surgery. Bariatric surgery is definitely a turning point in which *before* begins to morph into *after,* but you're the one who makes it happen. Surgery does not change your life; it gives you an opportunity to change your weight.

Surgical weight loss seemed like an excellent solution to my weight problem after seeing an ecstatic Carnie Wilson on the cover of *People* magazine in January 2001. The joy in her weight loss resonated with me at a time when my weight gain was making me miserable. Back then there weren't a lot of medical references that addressed the reality of long-term post-op life, which is why I began keeping my own files of notes, thoughts, and recipes to share with others. Over these years, we've watched Carnie struggle with alcohol and drugs—addiction transfers—and demonstrate emotional issues while appearing on a string of reality television shows that have placed bariatric patients in an unkind light. Without treating the underlying cause for compulsions, life continues along the same path. As for many post-ops, neither her joy nor weight loss was permanent.

In early 2012, Carnie announced that she had undergone a *second* bariatric surgery after gaining back substantial weight over a thirteen-year period. I'm hopeful that this time she accompanies her surgery with therapy, as it is probable that food is not her issue.

The more years that have passed since my 2001 RNY surgery, and the more I witness the problems surgery brings and how little people know about what they've done to their body, the more I back away from advocating this path. I prefer to focus on how those of us who have had bariatric surgery can make the most of the positive effects of our weight loss and can be proactive in preventing the negatives we now know come with it.

Bariatric surgery is not the fairy tale many believe it to be, and there's not a "happily ever after" ending for everyone. Self-induced and involuntary deficiencies are rampant, secondary medical issues such as hypoglycemia have not been addressed, patients with serious emotional disorders have surgery without diagnosis or therapy, and weight regain is the new emotional burden for patients too ashamed to go back to their surgeon.

My eyes have been opened to the high percentage of people who were morbidly obese because of emotional issues and undiagnosed personality disorders. For many, if not a majority, of those who are morbidly obese, it's not really about food. For years medical professionals have ignored the fact that morbid obesity is very often a symptom of a deeper emotional disorder. Surgery treats the indicator rather than the cause and removes the way people have survived by removing the ability to binge, gorge, soothe, and fill a void with food. After surgery, we are exactly the same person, except with a stomach that holds less food. People who have this surgery almost always need accompanying therapy—this is of crucial importance if this procedure is to continue.

I experienced an extreme instance when I befriended a bariatric patient whose outer shell hid emotional disturbances the likes of which I had never even considered. Innumerable incidents surrounded her that I now realize were staged, orchestrated, and embellished to the extent that I question everything that took place—medical emergencies and conditions, apartment floods and infestation, police run-ins, a near bathtub drowning, incoherent drunken calls, spousal abuse, dangerous dating scenarios, legal issues, garnishments, claims of being stalked, assertions of past lives and belief in the occult, the unfortunate death of a pet, veiled suicide references, and an eventual half-hearted suicide attempt.

I had no inkling these vignettes in all likelihood represented the life of someone with an *untreated* personality disorder. I unknowingly became part of the story by hiding the incidents; while I didn't know what to do, I surely didn't want anyone to think I had abandoned someone in such need. It escalated to the point where the constant tragedy in her life was dismantling mine; I felt trapped. But it was the only life this person knew; those with this condition crave the attention that a victim receives. I felt guilt yet relief when she moved on. I know I was not the first to experience the endless stream of catastrophic circumstances, and I'm certain they go on elsewhere with new and unsuspecting players.

Over these years, I have learned that weight-loss surgery is not a simple means to an end. From my wide vantage point over our surgical population, we have simply traded *what's in the box for what's behind the curtain,* without knowing what is behind it. In fact, even though we have an idea as to what is behind the inviting curtain and all it promises, very few people own their decision to make the trade.

When meeting someone who has had a *vertical sleeve gastrectomy*—or, even cuter, *the sleeve*—I've been sad to discover that they often don't know that most of their stomach has been removed. If you read about *sleeve* surgery, there's little if any direct reference to a healthy organ being dissected and removed from the body, so it's reasonable that a patient who is unfamiliar with medical terminology would not pick up on this. I do not think this procedure would be gaining in popularity if those having it knew exactly what it entailed.

One of the biggest problems is that no one knows the long-term implications of a twenty-year-old having most of their stomach removed. A well-known surgeon recently performed a sleeve procedure on a twelve-year-old family member and advocates such early interventions. Most twelve-year-olds are incapable of understanding the repercussions of cutting their own hair or leaving their cell phone at school—are they capable of living with the removal of 80 percent of their stomach *forever*?

Rather than encourage others to join in, I choose to work to help those who have already had surgery. This surgery is not easy— it takes dedication and serious life changes—and even when you're mindful of what you eat and how you live, there are likely effects in the future if not today. Before deciding on weight-loss surgery, read everything you can find from reputable, reasonable sources (noting that bloggers are not qualified medical sources unless they have a medical degree). Don't choose a surgeon because he works near your office or is listed at the top of the insurance book. Understand that you'll be giving up certain behaviors forever and must learn new ones and adhere to them for the rest of your life. Accept that what appears easy is often very difficult. Don't listen to advice from those who have not lived with bariatric surgery for at least ten years. And definitely find a therapist who can help you to discover why you're morbidly obese *before* you decide to have surgery.

Life after gastric bypass surgery is still an extraordinary journey, and after more than eleven years, I don't forget for even a minute that my happiness comes from the inside.

introduction

About a week before the life-altering bariatric surgery that would reduce my stomach to the size of a small egg, I found an envelope containing a folded, yellowed letter, neatly printed in pencil, in a box of family pictures. I had written it to my wonderful great-aunt Rose when I was six years old. Although it was precious to her, she had given it to my mother to save for me.

May 30, 1968

Dear Aunt Rose,

How are you and your family? We are all fine at home. This is my first letter to anyone. Mother helped me with the hard words. I get all A's on my report card. I am in the first grade. Grandpa said I could come to Florida with them next time to visit you. We will leave Johnny at home he's always crying for Mother . . . Dad is nice and skinny he lost 47 lbs of fat. Mom is skinny too. Johnny is skinny and I am getting tall. See you soon.

Love, Susan

I have always joked that I wasn't too heavy, I just wasn't tall enough; apparently I had already figured this out when I was in first grade. The words in the letter make me laugh, but clearly I was dealing with weight issues even as a six-year-old. I had analyzed my entire family and felt that I needed to justify myself; they weren't just thin, they were *skinny*. Did someone tell me not to worry about my weight because I would be getting taller sometime soon? Instead of pretending with my Barbie or playing on my swings, I was waiting to get tall.

I suffered from the usual assortment of childhood humiliations: innocently asking what the letters "OW" meant next to my second-grade weight of 91 pounds and having the school nurse loudly announce to a room full of my classmates that it stood for overweight; not being able to zip my powder blue one-piece gymsuit in Catholic grade school. Gym class was a source of terror throughout my school life in general, particularly the uneven parallel bars during a junior high gymnastics rotation. I stood in the back of the group afraid to even twitch; the sympathetic gym teacher mercifully lost track of me for a couple of weeks. There was a minor bright spot: two other fat girls in my class ranked even lower than I did since *they* couldn't throw or hit a ball, so at least I avoided the horror of being chosen last for teams. I overheard my best friend's older sister laughingly tell the cute new boy in town (and object of my summer crush) that I was a "baby blimp." At first I had no inkling that she was talking about me, but as the realization crept over me I felt the warm flush of shame as I stood in their kitchen. In fourth-grade English class, what were the odds that one of the spelling words of the day, *obese*, would correspond to my unfortunate choice of seat, where I had to stand up and correctly spell *and* use the word in a sentence? In grade school and junior high my father affectionately called me "Chubbette" and "Chubby." I still prefer to tell myself that it was simply his little term of endearment, and that he never would have used the pet name if he had thought he was hurting me, but in retrospect it does seem insensitive. These incidents are just a few that stand out in my mind; every fat person has his or her own repertoire of similar stories. I wouldn't want to go back in time to change them; who knows what I would be like today without these character builders?

I tried everything to lose weight. My mother took me to Weight Watchers meetings when I was 10. I have taken turns with Cambridge, Slim-Fast, Optifast, total food deprivation, Atkins, hormone injections, bizarre cabbage and banana régimes, hospital-supervised programs, and a nasty bout with bulimia in college while trying to keep off weight I had starved myself to lose for a spring-break trip. I would typically lose 20 pounds, then lose control and gain back 25 pounds. For most of my adult life, I have carried between 200 and 235 pounds on my medium 5-foot, 7-inch frame. Several years ago when I easily lost 32 pounds in two short months courtesy of the prescription weight-loss drugs fenfluramine and phentermine, commonly known as Fen-Phen, I thought these medications were finally going to be the thing that worked. Many of my friends were also taking this combination of pills that made it a breeze to push away the half-eaten plate of food, and we were a very happy group of losers. When the media storm about the side effects of fenfluramine and phentermine appeared, I decided that I was finished torturing myself with unhealthy diets. I convinced myself that being healthy and heavy were not mutually exclusive, and I could be both. I rationalized that I was fighting nature and that I should be happy the way I was meant to be. I always wore beautiful clothes and was meticulous about my hair and makeup. People knew I was competent and confident in business. I was happy and funny, I had an incredible husband and a great marriage, and now that I decided that I was not going to live within the restraints of dieting, I was finally free.

Over the next three years, I slowly but steadily ballooned to 278 pounds. I was now bursting out of 26/28, the largest size sold at Lane Bryant. The 3X sizes at Bloomingdale's were tight, and I became completely disgusted with what I had done to myself by eating whatever I wanted. My neck and chest were so large that I was having trouble breathing when I lay in bed. A custom, handmade sterling silver necklace that was a prize vacation purchase from Taxco, Mexico, now choked me. I couldn't even pretend I weighed less by creatively standing on one foot on the sweet spot on my scale. The cute, chubby little girl was now a morbidly obese 39-year-old woman; the "pretty face" was now distorted by fat into a face that I couldn't recognize in a mirror. For a few months I was actually thinking that the changes in the appearance of my face were a function of my approaching fortieth birthday rather than my approaching 300 pounds. When I started noticing that I didn't fit into booths at too many restaurants for it to be a coincidence, and I couldn't get my hair cut by John, my favorite stylist at In Sync because their zippered smocks didn't fit my increasing girth, I made more and more excuses to stay home. I spoke with my best friend, Ronni, on the phone almost daily, but didn't make the fifteen-minute trip to her home for over eight months. At my largest weight, I only left home to shop for groceries. I had few clothes that fit me, and I would stay in my silk bathrobe until late afternoon on most days. I was too humiliated by the smock situation to get my hair cut so I let it grow down to the middle of my back and rarely, if ever, made up my face anymore. I had so many "headaches" on days we were to attend parties and events that my husband suggested that I see a neurologist. As I got larger my world became very, very small.

In February 2001, I saw the image that changed my life: the newly svelte Carnie Wilson, Beach Boy Brian Wilson's daughter and member of the pop group Wilson Phillips, on the cover of *People* magazine. Carnie was standing with both of her legs in one leg of her "fat" jeans, wearing a petite, bright red peasant blouse, beaming with pure joy. I read that article over and over and was amazed by the weight-loss operation that I had previously only heard of in passing. The operation is called the Roux-en-Y Gastric Bypass procedure, commonly known as RNY. Even though the procedure was quite involved and the article stressed that it was major surgery, it didn't seem radical to me, since Carnie's procedure had been done laparoscopically through five tiny incisions. Carnie had learned about the procedure while appearing on Roseanne's show, when the comedian shared that she had lost almost 100 pounds after having had gastric bypass surgery the previous year. Carnie researched the details, made her decision, and, with the support of her family and friends, went ahead with the surgery, even broadcasting parts of the procedure on an Internet site. After losing almost half of her body weight, she was proudly showing off her physique in the pages of *People*.

I could relate to Carnie Wilson's story. As each of Wilson Phillips's hits was released with a video, Carnie was heavier and less prominently featured. She had a breathtakingly beautiful face, yet they tried to keep her body hidden and minimize her appearance in each song while Wendy Wilson, her extremely thin sister, and Chynna Phillips writhed around in lingerie. I was so embarrassed for her, and felt as if I were the only person who understood what she was going through. Seeing Carnie on that magazine cover and reading her story brought me to tears. I was so happy for her and for the hope that this surgery gave me. It was my defining moment: I realized how miserable I was at 278 pounds and decided that I had to do something about it.

I jumped on the Internet and started gathering every bit of information I could find about the Roux-en-Y Gastric Bypass operation. The stomach is reduced to a thumb-size pouch, from which the remainder of the stomach is divided with multiple rows of staples and permanently separated. The small intestine is cut about eighteen inches below the stomach, then pulled up and attached to the new small stomach pouch. The larger, lower portion of the stomach is bypassed, but it still provides digestive gastric juices for the small intestine. The small size of the pouch effectively stops the patient from eating too much at any given meal, while the bypassed intestine somewhat diminishes the ability to absorb the food that *is* eaten. A few ounces of food constitute a meal, and the sheer volume restriction on food intake is the first mechanism of weight loss. One or two small bites beyond satisfaction will create a stuffed feeling. A small bite beyond that will cause discomfort and nausea, and yet another small bite will cause pain and subsequent vomiting. The gastric reduction also works by creating satiety, the feeling of being comfortably full and satisfied. Filling the pouch with a small meal feels the same as if the whole stomach had been filled with a very large Thanksgiving feast. The pressure against the stomach walls triggers nerve signals that travel to the appetite center of the brain to give the feeling of satisfaction. Even though the portion size is small, there is no hunger and no feeling of having been deprived. People who have had this surgical procedure no longer live to eat, they eat to live. In other words, the gastric bypass surgery not only alters the anatomy for capacity, but also modifies how the brain's appetite center functions.

The best way to look at this procedure is to understand and visualize that the surgeon is creating a pouch, and this pouch is a tool to be used by the patient to control his or her weight. The surgery is not magic, and it can be a disaster if a patient expects the procedure to remove the weight automatically without changing his or her relationship with food. There is no jumping off the wagon for a holiday meal or special occasion. Bariatric surgery is not an easy way out for weight loss, as there are many potential trade-offs and changes in lifestyle. You have to accept the fact that you can *never again* gorge yourself on a multicourse meal of appetizer, salad, bread, Porterhouse steak with a loaded baked potato, cappuccino, and a crème brûlée. You have to deal emotionally with the fact that you can *never* eat all of anything, no matter how good it tastes. Physically, you can no longer eat more than a couple of ounces of tender filet mignon, two or three bites of a vegetable, and a small taste of the dessert. Early on, I just kept repeating my new mantra "Nothing tastes as good as thin feels!" Within a few months of surgery, it came true.

To be considered a candidate for the procedure, you must be clinically morbidly obese. Morbid obesity marks the point where

the disease begins to interfere with your basic physiological functions such as breathing, walking, and sleeping. It is defined as the
condition of weighing two or more times your ideal weight; however,
a more accurate indicator is having a Body Mass Index (BMI) of
40 (kg/m^2) or greater. BMI is a calculation that relates an individual's
weight to his or her height. The ideal BMI is between 19 and 25. If
you have a BMI of between 25 and 30, you are considered to be overweight. At a BMI of 30 or over, you are considered obese. A BMI of
40 or more indicates severe, or "morbid," obesity. Morbid obesity
increases the complications of pregnancy, surgery, and injuries, and
the incidence of breast and uterine cancers in women, prostate cancer
in men, and colon cancer in both. "Super morbid obesity" is defined
as 200 percent over ideal body weight, about 320 pounds for women
and 360 pounds for men; it exponentially increases the incidence
of disease, injuries, and early death. Gastric bypass surgery is only
presented as an option for those whose weight is high enough that
the medical risk of their obesity outweighs the risks of the procedure.

The RNY procedure is considered to be the most effective operation, offering the best combination of maximum weight loss with
minimum nutritional risk for the morbidly obese. The top bariatric surgeons agree that it is the best available operation at this time
in terms of *safety*, with less than a 0.5 percent mortality rate with
surgeons who are trained in this procedure, even taking into con-
sideration that these patients are high-risk operative candidates; *effec-
tiveness*, with patients averaging an 80 percent loss of excess weight
at one year; and *fewer undesirable side effects* for the patient, meaning
minimal vomiting, the ability to eat a wide selection of healthy normal
foods, and no chronic intestinal difficulties. More than 98 percent of
all weight-related health problems or comorbidities are relieved by
one year after the operation—usually within weeks.

The RNY gastric bypass procedure can be done using an open
technique gaining access to the abdomen through a single large mid-

line incision, or as a laparoscopic procedure. With laparoscopic surgery, the surgeons prepare the patient by inserting a series of tubes called *trocars* into tiny incisions. These tubes serve as channels through which the surgeon inserts a pencil-thin fiber-optic camera, which projects an image onto a television screen; a device to inflate the body cavity with gas to essentially float the organs apart; and long instruments with tips that cut, grip, and staple. It is an amazing and complex skill for a surgeon to master. The advantages to the patient are enormous: less pain, a shorter hospitalization, and a quicker return to normal life. Most of the post-op pain comes not from the organs operated on, but from the layers of skin, fat, and muscle tissue that were cut to gain access to them. Few surgeons are skilled in this highly specialized method of surgery, so finding a laparoscopic surgeon who performs the RNY gastric bypass operation can be a challenge in some parts of the country. Now that this procedure has grown in popularity, it is more important than ever to investigate the facts of this surgery: to become an expert on how your body will be affected by this operation, the risks and benefits as they pertain to you, and the background of the surgeon to whom you are entrusting your life. When flying on a commercial airliner you want a skilled and practiced pilot in the cockpit; when having this surgery, whether laparoscopic or open, you want a skilled and practiced surgeon with an established track record, who performs this procedure frequently.

After taking in mountains of information, I summoned my best friend, Ronni, and tentatively explained the surgery to her with the help of the popular website that had actually broadcast Carnie's surgery. We spent the entire day at my computer looking at before-and-after pictures, reading Carnie's narrative of her procedure, reading other peoples' accounts of their surgery, and discussing the actual procedure. I brought in a big basket of Doritos to snack on while we calculated our BMIs on the website. Size-four Ronni came in at a whopping BMI of 19 kg/m^2, while mine was almost 41 kg/m^2. Since I didn't have any medical conditions such as diabetes or hypertension to heighten my need for the procedure, my BMI had to be over 40 for me to even be considered for the surgery. Ronni pushed the Doritos toward me and said, "Here, eat these!" We laughed at the irony of my needing to maintain my pre-operative weight. It appeared that I was actually the perfect candidate for the RNY gastric bypass procedure. Gaining support from my wonderful husband, Ty, would be simple once I had the details ironed out.

I would not be alone in taking this permanent surgical step to solve my lifelong battle with weight. In 2001, more than 47,000 people had gastric bypass surgery. In 2002, more than 63,000 opted for the surgery, the number more than doubling since 1999. The 2011 figure of 225,000 bariatric procedures performed in the U.S. alone is staggering—world estimates now top over 350,000.

More people in the public eye are talking about their weight-loss surgery successes: opera star Deborah Voigt, blues legend Etta James, actress Roseanne Barr, *Real Housewives of New Jersey* daughter Lauren Manzo, insult comedian Lisa Lampanelli and her husband, Jimmy Big Balls, 1978's Buck Rogers TV hunk, Gill Gerard. Gospel singers Andrae and Sandra Crouch and showstopping singer and actress Jennifer Holliday can all be added to the list that already includes Star Jones, *American Idol* judge Randy Jackson, and author Anne Rice, who is best known for her best-selling novel *Interview with a Vampire*. They are on the heels of *Today* show weatherman and Food Network's Al Roker, who openly discussed his procedure after the nation witnessed his steady plunge from 320 to less than 190 pounds beginning in March 2002. Singer Ann Wilson, of Heart, underwent her bariatric procedure in January 2002 and for a time chronicled her progress on the same website that featured Carnie Wilson's surgical procedure. The front man for the band Blues Traveler, John Popper, went from over 420 pounds to a slim 185 after his RNY surgery in 2000. The NBC series *Ed* worked 500-pound actor

Michael Genadry's gastric bypass procedure into their story line for the 2003 season. Do you think that the Osbournes would have ever had a shot at MTV and mainstream stardom with a 250-pound, morbidly obese TV mom? Probably not! The now-diminutive Sharon Osbourne had her gastric procedure in 1999 and is enjoying incredible celebrity as the glue that holds this unconventional family together. Increasing numbers of public figures are announcing their successes with RNY surgery, thus creating an even bigger demand all over the country.

I needed to locate a bariatric surgeon to perform my surgery. I was very fortunate to find qualified laparoscopic bariatric surgeons where I live in South Florida. I scheduled my consultation with Dr. Carlos Carrasquilla for March 15, 2001. After completely disclosing all aspects of the procedure and giving me a thorough physical, Dr. Carrasquilla said that I was an excellent candidate for the laparoscopic procedure. I felt comfortable placing my future in his expert hands; his levels of confidence, skill, and experience were overwhelming and gave me the strength to make my final decision. With my approval to go ahead, his staff scheduled my surgery for June 11, 2001.

Now that I had a date for surgery, I had plenty of time to second-guess myself. My only hesitation was in regard to cooking and lifestyle. I absolutely love to cook and have been a "foodie" forever. I have always subscribed to *Gourmet* and *Bon Appétit* magazines. I have my TV tuned in to the Food Network at least six hours a day. I have aged balsamic vinegar in my kitchen along with chipotle peppers, wasabi powder, pure ancho chiles, tahini, fish sauce, twenty-eight bottles of hot sauce, a quart bottle of sriracha, a chunk of imported Parmigiano-Reggiano, and containers of oil-cured olives. My husband and I love to travel to Mexico, where I comb local markets in search of dried chiles, freshly made tortillas, and unusual fruit. Everywhere we go we sample local cuisine—ceviche, jerk pork, Pilsner beer, fiery salsas, hand-pressed olive oils, Black Forest ham, and cracked conch. Ty and I also collect agave tequila. On a trip to Germany, my goal was to track down a source of local homemade cherry liqueur, Kirschwasser. I love to make dinner and entertain at our home. I have baked magical candy-covered gingerbread houses for more than twenty-five years; it wouldn't be Christmas without them.

Food has always been a part of my life, and even though I was committed to changing my body and eating habits for better health, I didn't want to totally give up my lifestyle. Food is part of who I am. I didn't want to be thin and miserable; I didn't want to have to exist on special food while we traveled the world. I didn't want to be the freak eating the soup. So now that I had a surgical answer, I wanted to see if I could exist as an RNY gourmet.

I learned from other people who had had RNY surgery that we can eat normal food once we are past the first seven to eight months post-op, just in much smaller amounts. Everyone said their tastes and cravings had changed somewhat after surgery, and they now ate healthier foods. I discovered that those who had enjoyed hot, spicy, and bold flavors, like me, still enjoyed them post-op. I talked to people at their goal weight who had loved to cook before their surgery, and still loved to cook after their surgery. I learned from those who had undergone surgery that food had to be moist to be easy to eat and digest. In addition, sugar was no longer an option with the new configuration of our intestines, but with Splenda, NutraSweet, and other sugar-free innovations, I would be able to enjoy creative desserts and satisfy that occasional urge for a few bites of pie.

There was no reason that I wouldn't be able to travel, cook for my friends and family, and still enjoy cookbooks, Emeril Lagasse on television, and my subscription to *Gourmet* after my surgery. It was just going to take planning, experimentation, and dedication to a new way of eating.

the countdown
to june 11 begins!
pre-operative journal

May 26, 2001

I feel so weepy and emotional. I went to breakfast this morning with my husband, my father, and his wife, and I sat there staring at my plateful of scrambled eggs, fried potatoes, sausage, and bagel slathered with cream cheese; it made me feel so terrible about myself, I wanted to cry. I couldn't eat it. Lately, I analyze what is on my plate at every meal and think, "I will never eat this again." It is a very difficult feeling to deal with. Then five minutes later, I get angry with myself and think, "You have eaten enough in your life; get over it!" I regroup my thoughts and it is more like "I will never eat this much for one meal or on one plate again!"

June 5, 2001

My best friend, Ronni, and I checked out the surgical floor at Florida Medical Center. The fifth-floor bariatric suites appeared comfortable and clean. It made me feel so much better about the surgery looming before me. Everyone I have come in contact with at this hospital has been exceptional. When they perform a diagnostic test, the technicians are very professional and know what they are doing, and there is no confusion. You can feel so exposed and vulnerable in this setting, but the staff has given me even more confidence in my choice. The nurses took the time to talk to me and showed us around the floor, even taking us into one of the specially equipped bariatric rooms. I was surprised to see that this hospital has large leather recliners, and the beds have a steel frame canopy with a hanging bar you can use to help move yourself. I will be in a private room. Ronni will stay with me the first couple of nights since my husband can be pretty useless in medical situations, and I mean that in a loving way. I adore my husband, but after I had throat surgery two years ago, it took him entirely too long to figure out that my frantic hand gestures meant I desperately needed some water.

I have been comparing notes with people on the weight-loss surgery message boards and some of their hospitals and surgeons don't have scales capable of weighing them, or compression stockings to fit their large legs, or even hospital gowns for larger patients. I wonder why someone would choose a surgeon or a hospital that didn't make special accommodations for the comfort and safety of larger patients. More important, I wonder why a bariatric surgeon specializing in this procedure would not make sure that his or her hospital provided these items for their patients.

I only have a few days left to eat "big food," so tonight we are going out for pizza. Tomorrow, Ruth's Chris Steak House is on the calendar so that I can enjoy a final giant steak. I am 39 years old and I figure that I have eaten enough. I will be able to eat again, albeit in very small portions, but I will enjoy a few more days of shameless gluttony. I am scared, but on most days I can't wait to get rolling.

June 8, 2001

I am looking forward to being on the "losing" side of this surgery. Tonight, my husband went solo to a party we were invited to. The invitation touts that there will be a band with dancing, cocktails, and incredible food. I just didn't want to go. I am the biggest that I have ever been in my life, so of course my first thoughts were of my closet full of clothes too tight to wear. My newest size 26/28 Lane Bryant jeans are so tight that if that button on the waistband popped, the ricocheting metal could injure an innocent bystander. I can barely breathe while sitting down in them. My black knit twinset, the only acceptable item in my closet for a casual party, will make my makeup run in ten minutes flat in the humid June night air. Everyone will be running around in little tops and miniskirts and I would be the red-faced fat girl in the hot sweater and jeans. The clincher that cemented my decision to stay home was that it is a yacht christening party and I just know I would have been in an uncomfortable situation getting on and off the boat. I have already had a couple of embarrassing situations on friends' boats! Even when you can get on the boat, you have to worry about the tide changing. On one occasion a fairly easy two-foot jump down to the boat later became an impossible four-foot leap back up to the dock. I immediately recognized the problem at hand and watched in terror while everyone else seemed to fly effortlessly up to the dock aided by the helping hands of the uniformed boat valets. I tried to think of a reason to stay on the boat, but there was no way out. When my husband and a friend's husband realized that I was going to have difficulty getting up to the dock, they began to formulate a plan to help me. Then more of our friends became aware that there was a problem and got back on the boat to help. I found myself the sudden focus of attention while our well-meaning friends pulled and pushed me upward. As my feet landed on the dock, I tried to act nonchalant about whose hands had been on my butt, giving me that final boost. I suffered not only from embarrassment, but also large bruises on my arms and legs from the incident. This was supposed to be a fun end to a day of boating, but I remember it for the humiliation instead of the event we were celebrating.

Tonight, our dear friends giving the party will wonder where I am. I tried to beat it into my husband's head that information was to be given out strictly on a need-to-know basis. He is allowed to tell only those who asked that I am having my gallbladder removed on Monday. I am so sad to send him off by himself, but I have comfort in knowing that this is the last time.

June 10, 2001

I am spending this last night before my surgery reading the online journals of people who have had weight-loss surgery. There are so many women who are the same age, height, and weight as I am, that I am able to get a pretty reasonable picture of what to expect. After reading at least 100 stories and clicking on hundreds of before-and-after pictures, I am at peace with the whole thing. I have eaten my last meal of Sunday morning blueberry pancakes drenched with butter and drowning in real Vermont maple syrup. Now I can only have clear liquids until midnight and then nothing by mouth. I feel as if I am in a plane with my parachute carefully packed.

june 11, 2001 . . . my post-op life begins!

post-operative journal

June 22, 2001

My surgery was much tougher than I expected. Other patients from the same day were in and out in three days; my procedure took longer than usual and involved a great deal of tugging and pulling to get my parts where they needed to be. If I hadn't had such an experienced surgeon, my laparoscopic RNY would have turned into an open RNY. I am lucky that Dr. Carrasquilla has had other tough cases. This proves my theory that you don't need a great surgeon for a routine procedure, you need one in case your procedure produces the unexpected. In addition, my intestines didn't quite "wake up" from the surgery for a few days, creating lots of trapped gas. So, after the first days of feeling as if I had been hit by a large truck, I quickly recovered and spent the rest of my hospital time feeling fine (considering that I had just had my guts rearranged), but waiting to blow out the gas! The nurses not only took great care of my physical needs, but also knew how to handle my vulnerability. I had a longer hospital stay than most and they knew how disappointed I was about it. The nurses couldn't have been more wonderful; I just didn't expect to stay with them for nine days for a laparoscopic procedure.

This is my third night at home. I am still very uncomfortable with these staples—I am afraid they will catch on something. My stomach is swollen and somewhat bruised. I look like a manatee with my huge, bloated belly. The five cuts scattered across my belly are a strange sight. I am scheduled to have the staples removed tomorrow. The water and broth that I am constantly sipping is going down easily. I have not had any trouble at all with nausea or vomiting. I have an overall feeling of fullness and although I am not hungry, I made myself eat several small bites of food each day since I am sure that my body needs protein after all it has been through. A protein shake is easy for me to eat and takes a good half an hour to consume. The creamy, cold, banana protein shake I make every morning makes me feel very full. I sit at my computer sipping my shake instead of coffee while I read my e-mail. I can feel it trickling down into my stomach as the coldness spreads downward. How odd. Cold and thick seems to work better than a thin liquid shake.

My family is coming over for a barbecue this weekend. I plan on making some pinto bean puree, a large salad, and grilled turkey burgers; a feast for all and I can eat a small portion of beans, since I am restricted to eating soft foods. I am beginning to understand the lifestyle changes I will need to make.

June 25, 2001

I am healing very well and I feel great. My only complaint is that I have one spot that pulls and burns when I get out of bed from a flat position. I am still eating pureed foods like egg custard and sugar-free pudding, and I have not had any problems at all. I have a second protein shake in the afternoon since I need the protein to heal. If I can just eat small portions of normal foods, this will be easy. I had my staples removed on Friday and it didn't even pinch. It seems that the holes from the staples are worse than the incisions. I have seven little cuts, actually five little cuts and two drain holes . . . twenty-one staples in all but nothing that some Neosporin won't heal. I was afraid to get on the scale at the doctor's office because of all the bloat I still have in my belly, but the surgical assistant cajoled me and I have lost 16 pounds. Ta da! I was shocked.

July 7, 2001

So here I am at 25 days post-op, and just getting back to feeling good again! The food situation is revealing itself. At first, I didn't understand why I didn't really get a full feeling with very soft foods. I was worrying that my pouch may have been fashioned in too large a size. Now that I am eating more solid items, feeling full sneaks up on me! I measure out my little portions of food for my plate and sometimes I can get only halfway through those small amounts. I am through before I am ready to be! Soups, custards, and tuna salad taste the best and go down easily. I didn't understand other people talking about foods being moist when I was pre-op, but the other day when I made turkey burgers on the grill, after three small bites I felt as though I had eaten three pounds of burger and it was all backed up in my chest. The feeling was very unpleasant, so I pushed food around on my plate so my family didn't question me. I don't want my surgery to put me in the spotlight, which is why I had everyone over for dinner in the first place. Good thing I made pinto bean puree with a little light sour cream and cheddar on top; it was delicious. My favorite egg salad doesn't taste good anymore. Oddly enough I am finding that I don't care what or if I am eating. I never thought that this would happen to the Food Network's number one viewer.

My husband is talking about taking a trip to the Mirage in Las Vegas. I had to laugh because my first thought was that my breakfast days of prime rib, jumbo shrimp, and bagels smeared with cream cheese and piled high with smoked salmon are over! I can't believe that my first thoughts are of the food I will be missing. It goes to show you that it takes a while for your head to catch up with your body after this procedure. Then I had wonderful thoughts of being able to buy a gorgeous blouse or pair of pants in one of those expensive "thin people's" boutiques, or being able to buy the David Yurman bracelet that I want with my winnings and not having to settle for the only one that fits my large wrist. On this next trip things will be different! I told Ty that I will play blackjack in the seat next to him because now I won't keep bugging him that it is time for supper!

July 12, 2001

I am one month post-op! I never thought that I would feel this good so quickly. I walk on the treadmill six days a week and my weight loss is keeping me going. I went to put on a pair of jeans yesterday and they fell off my hips! I couldn't believe it. I had so much swelling and bloat in my lower belly that I couldn't even button the jeans two weeks ago. When I stepped on the scale at the surgeon's office, the nurse put the big weight on 200. I cringed and told her she needed to move it to 250, but then when she slid the small weight over, it balanced at 47. I couldn't believe that I only weigh 247! That is 31 pounds in one month. No wonder my jeans were so loose.

My husband got me going this morning when I put on my baggy jeans. He told me to go to my closet and put all my clothes that are the same size as the baggy jeans in a bag and take them to the church thrift store, since I will never be big enough to wear them again for the rest of my life. How is that for a happy reality moment? I have cleaned out my drawers and my closet and found all kinds of great outfits that will fit again soon! I am thrilled. I am officially happy to have had this surgery. Until now, I vacillated between regret and cautious optimism.

I have been eating fish almost every night without any trouble. Grilled salmon, baked tilapia, or sautéed shrimp, with low- or no-fat sauces for the fish and a very small portion of the vegetables I made for the family. My favorite is mango salsa. I mix finely diced mango with lime juice, cilantro, red onion, and Tabasco, then add a tablespoon of olive oil, salt, and pepper. It can moisten a piece of fish or even roasted turkey breast, but at this point the fish is much easier for me to digest. I tried a bit of grilled chicken and it didn't seem to go down as well, giving me indigestion and an uncomfortable overstuffed feeling after a bite or two. I will stick to fish and shrimp.

I find that a protein shake is great for breakfast and gives me a much-needed 30 grams of protein. I can see that with as little as I can eat for a meal, I will always have to be conscientious about taking in enough protein. Zero Carb Isopure Creamy Vanilla works—with a small piece of banana, skim milk, and some ice, it is tasty and smooth to sip.

As far as food—still no nausea or problems. When I woke up from surgery I *never* thought I would ever feel this good again! The scars on my stomach are fine pink dashes and will be gone by the end of the summer. I am slowly melting.

July 23, 2001

I invited my dad and his wife, Diane, for the first spaghetti and meatball Sunday dinner since my operation. It's tough for Italians to go without sauce for six weeks! I made little meatballs so I could have two of them, and I ate two pieces of ziti. I put lots of sauce on top so it was soupy.

The problem came later on when we broke out the Pepperidge Farm cake that my Dad so thoughtfully brought for my husband's birthday. I cut the cake into huge pieces so everyone else would eat it all. I never realized how tough it is to *not* lick your fingers when you cut a layer cake. But I resisted the urge. Actually the prospect of getting sick with "dumping syndrome" in front of everyone in my living room kept my frosting-filled fingers out of my mouth! I had an

Eskimo Pie sugar-free fudge pop and although it was chocolaty, it certainly was not Pepperidge Farm cake. Oh well, I am sure it didn't taste as good as thin will feel.

July 30, 2001

Well this is day 49 post-op and my *only* complaint is that I still can't sleep on my stomach. The pain between my belly button and the left incision has finally gone away. I stopped walking for a few days, stopped bending over, stopped twisting my hips, and stopped doing everything that made the pain stab. The doctor checked me out and said it wasn't a hernia, just the nerve endings shooting off until the muscle mends. Some people are just sensitive and have more pain. The lower left incisions are commonly the cause of some distress since this is the site through which most of the surgery is done, and therefore has more muscle tearing and stretching. A few days ago, I woke up and the pain was gone. I have resumed walking again.

Got on the scale and in 49 post-op days I have lost 43 pounds. Yesterday, when I ate too fast, I threw up. It is actually better described as regurgitation. It was the same chewed-up mouthful of food I had earlier eaten, but since I do not have stomach acid it was not vile. I had better pay attention and eat slowly. I recall my surgeon explaining that our stomach configuration is like the drain in a sink; if you turn on the water slowly, the water smoothly flows down the drain, but if you turn on the water full force, the drain backs up.

I feel fantastic. I have so much energy. I am excited about finding clothes in my closet that fit me again and even more excited about taking my old big clothes to the church thrift store. My goal is to be down 50 pounds in 60 days and I believe that I will make it.

August 8, 2001

I made it through my first post-op sushi experience. My very first *restaurant* experience, actually. We were out having cocktails with friends (I had my bottle of water) and the idea came up to grab some sushi. I was a little nervous but figured I could wing it.

I ordered four thin pieces of tuna sashimi, just the fish slices without rice, and a Florida hand roll: sliced scallops baked with scallions, fish roe, and spicy Japanese mayonnaise rolled into a cone of seaweed. I picked the scallops out of the cone; the sauce made them easy to eat. I gave Ty two pieces of my tuna, since I was getting full. All in all, a great restaurant experience! Dr. Carrasquilla was right; I have become a cheap date. Our usual $80 sushi tab was just $35 tonight.

August 13, 2001

I don't have an official reading on my doctor's scale until August 21, but unofficially I have lost 53 pounds in nine weeks! I am so excited and I can't believe how fast I am dropping in size. I had better wear some of my smaller clothes quickly or I will miss the opportunity. Even though it seems I am not losing as much weight as in the very beginning, I am losing more inches than before. I have lost four sizes.

I am still preparing dinners for my friends and family, who still love my cooking and haven't noticed that everything is lower in fat and carbs. I am still a great cook!

September 16, 2001

I ate some crab sticks for lunch this afternoon and have felt sick ever since. About an hour after I ate them I started feeling terrible. Ty sells real estate and we were showing a million-dollar home to customers when I had to drop back from the group to throw up in the master bathroom. When I lifted the seat on the commode, I realized that the water wasn't hooked up yet. I ran outside and spit up into the bushes. I was so embarrassed. I spent about 40 minutes avoiding my husband and the clients as they toured the home, so they wouldn't see me retching in the shrubbery. I only ate three pieces of the stuff and threw up a much greater volume than I consumed. I finally made it home and collapsed on my bed. I tried drinking some water, but that flew out too. I haven't eaten anything that could have blocked my opening. This was not a good day. Note: Susan will not be eating crappy surimi imitation crab ever again!

September 30, 2001

I am so happy about this surgery; it is the best thing I could have done for myself. I am addicted to my scale and weigh myself every morning. I am poised at breaking the 200 mark, but cannot imagine being less than 200 pounds.

I am adding a wider range of soft foods, in small portions. Best of all, eating in restaurants isn't the problem I thought it would be. I went to a birthday party at a restaurant last night and I didn't order my own food, since the portions were so large. I just asked Ronni if I could share hers. Her fish entrée arrived and there were four huge planks of blackened grouper. She would never have been able to eat all of it, and even together we didn't finish the plate. Another friend had an Asian chicken salad and I had some of her greens. It is amazing how everyone is so interested in my surgery, encouraging me to eat off their plates instead of ordering my own. Everyone is paying attention to my new eating habits, watching how little I eat, observing how small I cut my pieces and how long I chew my food. Nothing tastes as good as being thinner feels. I can finally say that with confidence. My clothes are hanging on me. I just bought two shirts in size

18 that are on the verge of being too big for me! I should have ordered a 16 for sure.

October 11, 2001

I just walked in from a wonderful evening out and had to sit down and write about the unabashed happiness I am experiencing. For those of you struggling with your decision to have the surgery, and those of you who have just had their surgery and are struggling with the first few weeks: it all gets so much better! My four-month post-op anniversary is tomorrow and I have lost 79 pounds as of this morning.

Friends who have a membership in the Tower Club, an exclusive private dinner club in downtown Fort Lauderdale, invited us to dinner. The view of the ocean, Intracoastal Waterway, and city lights was breathtaking, the room beautiful, and the staff superlative. The food was excellent. I ate an incredible dinner and stayed within my guidelines.

Cocktails were served in the lounge, along with hors d'oeuvres. I had an imported mineral water served in a champagne glass so it would appear that I was having a cocktail. We were then seated in the main dining room with a 360-degree bird's-eye view of the city and ocean. A small square of pâté on rye toast was served as a palate teaser while we looked at our menus. I only nibbled a corner of the pâté, and didn't touch the hot roll placed on my bread plate. I shared a pear and blue cheese salad with raspberries and baby greens with Jayne. I ate slowly and chewed well but consumed less than half of the half portion I was served. Then a palate cleanser of fresh raspberry sorbet was served in a beautiful etched glass dish; much as I would have liked to taste it, I passed, since I was not sure of the sugar content. I knew that sugar could make me sick with the new configuration of my stomach and intestines, and didn't want to test my limits.

My entrée soon followed: a whole Dover sole, boned tableside and placed on a platter with a swirl of potato puree, baby green beans, and baby yellow squash. The fish was so fresh and the light lemon, butter, and caper sauce was delicious. I ate most of one half of the fish fillet since protein comes first, skipped the potato carbs, and ate a couple of green beans. The dessert cart was presented. My heart sank as the first plate was set down with a large hunk of a chocolate raspberry cheesecake torte with raspberry coulis, then a slice of mango cake with fruit puree and cream decorating the large platter, and the signature crème brûlée. I sighed and told my friends to order the first one so I could watch them enjoy it. The waiter picked up on my sad tone and asked me why none of the selections pleased me. I stumbled for a second and then mumbled as a cover that I was a diabetic. Without missing a beat he smiled and told me the pastry chef is famous for his sugar-free chocolate chip cheesecake, or would be happy to make me a dish of mixed berries with a sugar-free Romanoff sauce. He said they would serve a sliver, a slice, or a slab. I asked for a sliver of the sugar-free cheesecake and a cappuccino. I tasted my sugar-free cheesecake and was in heaven. It was delicious, but even though it was sugar-free I ate only three small bites since I was full. I sampled one of Ty's blackberries with a dab of the Romanoff sauce. I sipped my cappuccino and enjoyed the rest of the evening smiling broadly, knowing that I had just enjoyed a fabulous dinner that would not prevent me from losing my eightieth pound on my four-month post-op anniversary tomorrow! I love what this surgery has done for me and I love my life, my friends, my husband, the way I feel, my new slimmer body in my newly fitting narrow black pants and favorite chartreuse and black lace blouse. Life is excellent and it will get even better.

October 20, 2001

I am getting ready for a 1950s party that we have been invited to attend this evening. It isn't too often that I wear short socks and a skirt that twirls in the air when I spin. I have a custom-made, thick pink felt skirt, appliquéd with a black fuzzy poodle with a rhinestone collar and braided leash, a black twin sweater set, a sheer pink scarf to fasten my ponytail, rolled down bobby socks, black and white Bass saddle shoes, and my husband's 1958 class ring on a gold chain for the finishing touch. I splurged and ordered the stiff full crinolines to wear under my skirt. When I put the crinolines on, my skirt is so big I can't get though the door. How am I going to go to the bathroom in this outfit without dunking my skirt in the toilet? I wouldn't have considered going to this party if I hadn't lost this weight. I would have been much too self-conscious to squeeze my 300-pound body into a big pink skirt.

Other than Ty drinking too much tequila and acting like a frat boy in front of all our friends, the party was great. I found it was very difficult to find something to eat. The '50s theme featured carhop food. There was a hot dog cart, a large grill with genuine White Castle burgers sizzling away, French fries bubbling in submerged baskets, a cotton candy machine, a popcorn machine, all set up in the enormous courtyard driveway. Then dinner was served in the "malt shop": meat loaf, macaroni and cheese, green beans, and corn. There was a soda fountain set up with sundaes and milk shakes, hmm . . . still nothing for me to eat. I tried to eat a White Castle burger but it was too greasy. The music was great, and I easily had the most authentic outfit at the party. No one else had crinolines— they really made my outfit. What fun it is to dance and twirl around and spin and jitterbug. What a fun party. Losing this weight is fantastic. I felt so free to dance and have fun. I could tell that several of our friends noticed that there was something different about me and made a point of mentioning that I looked great, but no one attributed it to losing weight. I am not discouraged by this as these aren't people who see me often enough to notice 80 pounds.

November 3, 2001

Last night we celebrated Ronni's birthday. The plan was for a few friends to meet at her home and drive to a special restaurant for dinner. When I arrived at her home I discovered that the plan had changed, and her cool and stylish mom, Joyce, had hired a stretch limousine to take all of us to The Blue Door at the Delano in South Beach, Miami. Dealing with this food challenge was a real test for me. I was excited at the idea of eating in this well-known restaurant, but I feared that I would struggle with the restrictive component of my surgery. Would the happiness I would derive from sitting at the table in a smaller size be enough to compensate for not being able to finish my heaping plate?

What a breathtaking entrance and lobby! Soaring ceilings with long, sheer, flowing white drapes billowing in the ocean breeze, blurring the definition between inside and out. There were walls but it seemed as if we were outside with the night air and fresh breeze blowing through the hotel. All four walls of the dining room were lined with the same gossamer white draperies, and all the beautiful waiters were dressed from head to toe in white. The only decorations were etched Venetian mirrors and a large mirrored pedestal in the center of the dining room with a hundred ivory candles of different sizes and heights flickering in the gentle wind. It was so beautiful and elegant, a total thrill to the senses.

Dinner was sublime. I shared a salad of baby greens, pears, and prosciutto with mango-lime vinaigrette with Ronni. I had a tiny taste of a blue cheese Napoleon and of a crab and avocado terrine that were as delicious as they were beautiful. These plates of food were too much for words—each was an edible work of art. I ordered an entrée of lightly sautéed lobster on a crisp risotto cake with a passion fruit–herb reduction, braised baby bok choy, and cashews. It was very tender and really scrumptious. I was able to eat about half of the tail.

Dessert was going to be difficult, because they did not have any diabetic, sugar-free, or plain fruit desserts. I was going to have to implement the tiny taste method. Joyce had a mango baked Alaska: mango and passion fruit sorbet on an almond biscuit covered with meringue, baked, and placed in the center of a huge pool of mango-passion fruit sauce with raspberry sauce swirls and chopped mangos. It wasn't overly sweet, so I had two very small bites. Ronni had a melted chocolate cake with pistachio ice cream, one of those perfect little cakes that are hot liquid chocolate inside when you cut into it. I didn't taste that one at all because it looked too dangerously sweet. Another friend had a mascarpone cheesecake, a super-rich individual round with mango sauce on the plate and a burnt sugar crust. One small bite was divine. I also had a cappuccino with skim milk foam that was served in a beautiful oversized cup and saucer.

I'm thrilled that this surgery still allows me to do such great things and live life. Before my bariatric surgery, I was very worried that I would never be able to enjoy incredible evenings out, but it isn't a problem at all since there is always at least one good choice on any menu. I can't wait until I am even thinner in a few months! I feel so healthy and strong and full of energy.

Tomorrow is part two of the birthday celebration. Ronni, Joyce, and I are spending the day at the Hilton Bonaventure Spa. Six months ago I never would have considered something like this. I would have made excuses to avoid going. I am going to be one smooth and radiant chick when I get finished tomorrow.

November 5, 2001

Five years ago the owner of the company I was working with rewarded me with a full day at this same spa. I was humiliated within
fifteen minutes of my arrival when the spa's robe didn't close and
the staff acted as though no one had ever had this problem before. It
was one of the worst days of my life. I spent every second not knowing whether to burst into tears or run out of there, but I had to stay
since another manager had also been given the day off to use our
motivational gift.

This time it was different. I was of normal size, comparatively
speaking, and I wasn't embarrassed to disrobe alongside my slender
friend Ronni in the women's locker room. She looked at me and
couldn't believe how much smaller I was already. When I took the
thick white terry robe off the hanger of my locker and slipped it on, it
was the moment of truth. The robe had plenty of overlap and felt soft
and luxurious; I was so very happy.

We got our slippers and strolled into the salon for our pedicures.
Next was my body treatment. When I walked into the wet treatment
room, the clinician handed me a paper and elastic thong panty to put
on—eeeeeeeeeeekkkkkkk! Scary to have to wear a thong—but it fit! I
had to hang up my robe and lie facedown on the plastic-lined padded
table while two clinicians with loofah mitts exfoliated the back of my
body with the most delicious-smelling almond oatmeal scrub. My
first thought was of how many carbs must be in the thick mixture! I
had to flip over onto my back so they could scrub my front, and then
flip over once again, no problem. Then they smoothed jet black Dead
Sea mud all over me. I was wrapped in plastic sheets, then enveloped
in thick heated padded blankets. The lights were dimmed and the
women told me to relax for 40 minutes. Wrapped in this warm co-
coon, I thought about how different this spa trip was turning out;
I gently fell in and out of a light sleep while I felt the warm mud

squishing as I moved slightly. One woman unwrapped me while the other turned on the shower. When I stepped from the shower I was handed two towels. I fashioned one for my hair into a turban and wrapped the second around me without thinking. Then it dawned on me that I had just wrapped a towel around myself! Another thrilling moment and it wasn't even a large towel. I was glowing, and not just from my mud treatment.

Now it was time for my facial. An older woman with a European accent came out and called my name. I followed her into the dimly lit room and reclined on the padded table. She put a bolster under my knees and a pillow under my head. A moist cloth was placed over my eyes and I was sprayed with a cool mist. My facial was incredible. She massaged the muscles in my neck and face and it felt so good I thought I was going to pass out.

I never dreamed in June that less than five months later I would actually have a great day at this spa. I started out a little nervous but left feeling soft and smooth and confident! I can't wait to go again.

November 27, 2001

We just returned home from Georgia after celebrating a Southern Thanksgivin' with my husband's kinfolk. As I had anticipated, Georgia food was not good for me. The turkey was so overdone that it was like sawdust when you chewed it. Their family recipe for gravy involves cooking lard with flour and milk then adding chopped hard-boiled eggs and chicken meat to the concoction. There was no way that I could moisten my food with this chunky slurry. I sneaked some of the drippings from the roasting pan into a cup and heated them in the microwave to pour over a few shreds of dark meat. I couldn't eat the sweet potato casserole made with brown sugar, marshmallows, and pecans. The vegetables were all cooked with fatback but they were at least tender, so I ate a few green beans.

I couldn't eat the ham because it was too solid in consistency and dripping with cane syrup. It was a very difficult food day for me, and I ended up throwing up every bit that I ate. The only thing that was soft and easy for me to eat was the sugar-free pumpkin pie that I had baked at home and taken with us. To make it worse, everyone ate the leftovers for the next three days so I basically existed on my pie and coconut protein bars. I did wish that I could eat, but there will be other holidays when I will be able to prepare the food.

I felt so thin the entire time I was there and I knew I would lose a few pounds this Thanksgiving. Many of Ty's relatives didn't know how huge I was just five months ago and all they talked about was how pretty I was. It is hard to think of yourself as pretty when you were close to 300 pounds and you still have the fat clothes in your closet to remind you. I even asked Ty if the mirror in our bedroom was off and did it make him look thinner too. He laughed and said that the reflection was true and that I did look thin. When I weighed myself this morning I realized why I felt so thin; I am down to 180! I cannot believe it. I guess the plateau that had me bummed the last three weeks is over. The amazing part is that four pounds at this weight make a huge difference!

Ty's very petite and beautiful daughter, Dione, taught me a lesson about my changing body image. She weighs just 110 pounds and easily slips into a size four, but her lower stomach is loose and stretched out after having three children. It made me very happy to see this! I don't mean that in a bad way because I love her dearly. We were talking about my weight loss and I told her about the embarrassing flap of skin squishing out over the waistband of my jeans, when she showed me her stomach. Seeing her belly and knowing how she felt made a big difference in how I feel about myself during this transitional weight-loss period. We women are all too tough on ourselves, no matter what our weight.

January 1, 2002

Wow . . . what a year for me! From a bursting-at-the-seams 278 to a still-shrinking 172 pounds in less than seven months. I never would have guessed it if you had asked me last January first, since I had not even thought about RNY surgery as a possibility at that point. I feel fantastic and I am gaining more confidence every day as I evolve.

My husband is giving me some trouble; he is having a hard time adjusting to the fact that I want to go out with my girlfriends to lunch and spend time doing things. I was essentially a shut-in by choice the last two years. I didn't get dressed up every day or do my hair or even put on makeup. I had such a poor self-image that I didn't care anymore and made excuses to not take part in life. I talked to my girlfriends on the phone but didn't go anywhere with them. I hadn't stepped into a mall in over three years! Ty got used to this and since we work from home, he liked having me around 24/7. So now that his butterfly is flitting around and he's competing for my time, he is getting his back up. I am sure this has happened with many other women, and men, who have had this surgery. It may be amplified in my case, since my husband is 22 years older than I am. I met him when I was 21 but we have been together for almost 20 years. We have never had age issues and I don't think that this is necessarily the problem, but he keeps saying he knows how men are. I keep reminding him that I am not hanging out in bars and clubs, I am going to the mall or my girlfriends' houses. Things got a little tough around Christmas but seem better this week. I was spending a lot of time at Ronni's house baking cookies and gingerbread houses for Ty's grandchildren. Now that the holidays are over I am sure that things will improve. Those of you who are married should prepare for changes in your spouse's attitude—it is inevitable. We have been together so long I just have to remind him that I am not going anywhere. Ty is a very exciting person to be with, always spontaneous and adventurous, and now that I am not dragging my feet and sabotaging his plans, we will enjoy many more years together.

February 8, 2002

The needle on the scale has not moved since Christmas. *This* is a plateau, not what people perceive as a plateau when they are ten weeks post-op. I am in my third week of a serious weight-lifting and aerobic exercise program, so I am fine with not having lost any more weight. I keep telling myself that just 12 months at 2 pounds a month will get me where I want to be. I am in perfect health.

Before I had my RNY surgery I had serious thyroid problems. In 1999 I had half of my thyroid removed when it was discovered that the gland was wrapped around my trachea and literally choking me. When it was removed, the surgeon found it had grown under my collarbone and into my chest cavity. Two weeks before my RNY surgery last June, my endocrinologist here in Fort Lauderdale wanted me to go off my Synthroid and have a nuclear test on a couple of nodules she had spied on my latest thyroid ultrasound. If I had gone off my medicine, I would have been forced to cancel my gastric bypass surgery. After much thought, I decided that I would deal with my thyroid later and go ahead and have my RNY surgery. So now that I am eight months post-op gastric bypass surgery, I went ahead and scheduled a guided needle biopsy of those pesky nodules my endocrinologist wanted to have a look at. I was on the table; the ultrasound technician called in another technician, then another technician, and finally the radiologist. They were all taking turns on me with the rollerball probe to pinpoint what to biopsy before they inserted the needle. I was terrified, worrying about what they might have seen that was devastating enough to keep all four gathered around the screen. They didn't see anything; there weren't any nodules. After losing all this weight and being on the same Synthroid dosage for these months, the nodules had disappeared! The radiologist was pleased to tell me that they couldn't locate any nodules in my neck to biopsy. The weight of the world was off my shoulders.

February 13, 2002

I have a girlfriend, Stephanie, who was the same pre-operative size as I was, and who had her RNY procedure one week before I did. We were both unhappy about our clothes hanging from us as if they belonged to someone else, and decided to go on a shopping excursion to Macy's at Palm Beach Gardens Mall on Sunday. I do have to admit: it was one of my most inspired shopping trips to date. We had at least 100 pieces of clearance-priced clothing in those dressing rooms; then we swapped what didn't fit or what we didn't like by tossing it over the top of each other's booth, laughing the entire time. She is more of a 12 and I am a too-tight 12 and a better 14, so we are fairly compatible for shopping. Let me inquire, though, just when was it decided that pants didn't need to come up past your belly button? I guess Lane Bryant didn't jump on *that* bandwagon. I had two epiphanies in that dressing room in a pair of size 12 DKNY pants as my loose belly fat spilled out and over the top of the incredibly low-riding pants: first, that I didn't like this fashion trend at all and, second, that I am not as thin as I thought I was! The pants fit but it seemed like there were four to six inches of vital fabric missing. Nope, the 14 didn't have any more coverage, although it didn't seem to squeeze my Jell-O–like abdomen quite as obscenely. Hello fellow shoppers? Given that this *is* Palm Beach, would anyone in this dressing room have the number of a plastic surgeon handy?

We hit the food court and split a tuna wrap, picking apart our food like four-year-olds, leaving the remains of our forage for protein on the tray. On the way past the Häagen-Dazs booth, Stephanie shared a bariatric secret with me. She asks for a sample of the Häagen-Dazs sugar-free soft yogurt and then savors the little free sample cup since she is now satisfied with just a taste. Not this time, though. We shared a small cup of the creamy chocolate-vanilla swirl and I couldn't believe it wasn't full of sugar—it really tasted too good to be sugar-free. We sat on the edge of a planter and enjoyed our little treat.

Shopping is much better now than when I followed Ronni around the stores and suffered the embarrassment of leaving the dressing room to try to locate a size four from the rack before the genius salesgirls tracked me down to ask me what I was looking for. I always imagined they were laughing at me, thinking to themselves that nothing in the store would fit someone my size.

February 24, 2002

When you lose a lot of weight and get your life back, there are lots of crazy things you do that just a short time earlier you would never even have thought of! My husband and I bought a Harley-Davidson V-Rod motorcycle two weeks ago and leased a condo on the ocean in Daytona Beach for Bike Week! I am amazed at how much fun my life is now—or maybe it just really sucked when I weighed almost 300 pounds. If you had told me last year that I would be going to Daytona to party for Bike Week, I would have laughed at you. This is my first big adventure in at least two years, since we stopped vacationing when I was at my heaviest. I somehow squashed our sense of adventure by always making the dates inconvenient. I just manipulated our schedules in order to not get into uncomfortable situations on planes, in restaurants, amusement parks, and rental cars, and in boutiques with narrow aisles. I was hiding while life passed me by. I am ready to start living again and this time I am out of the chute on the back of a Harley! My family is beginning to worry about me.

March 9, 2002

We are home from Daytona and I had an amazing time! This was a week of fun, shiny chrome motorcycles, incredible people, and excellent food too! I can easily say that there was no way I could have ever done any of this without this surgery and losing all of that fat! I feel the urge to hug and kiss Dr. Carrasquilla right now. I didn't realize it, but our last few vacations were terrible. I felt so self-conscious about my appearance and tried so hard to avoid fat situations, that it made the trips into one-week-long arguments.

From day one I was perched on the back of that Harley looking cool in my black leather jacket and loving the attention that our motorcycle was getting and the attention that we were getting! I do have to say we had really great outfits. I love this biker thing, as it combines a sport with fashion and makeup! I even bought a pair of black leather chaps, so now I am an official badass! The big joke among riders is the mystique of women wearing their chaps with just a thong. I really laughed at that one, as I definitely am not that kind of girl, but maybe I'll change my mind when I am 125 pounds.

We had a condo on this trip and I cooked big breakfasts for everyone each morning so I usually had an egg and some ham or sausage with a bite or two of biscuit. Lunch was a protein bar or some rolled up sandwich meat, and supper was shrimp or fish and a couple of raw oysters. I ate raw oysters all week; they were so good and easy to eat! I did have a few of what I would consider cheats during my week. I sampled a margarita that was made with fresh lime so there was no sugar or sweetened mix added. I drank half of that and got tipsy very quickly. I tasted a rum and Diet Coke and decided it was a horrible-tasting drink. I ate a few Fritos after my picnic lunch of half a turkey sandwich and threw up everything in the Kennedy Space Center parking lot. I had a few bites of the best Key lime pie I had ever tasted three nights in a row at an unbelievable fish camp restaurant. I had a spectacular time on this vacation and I even lost some weight. My butt felt smaller on that seat and my jeans are baggier because I managed to lose three pounds.

March 23, 2002

I am nine months, ten days post-op and we went to a surprise birthday party for a friend tonight! No one from this group of friends had laid eyes on me since I was three months post-op and modeling my 1950s skirt and crinolines, so my weight loss hadn't necessarily smacked everyone in the face that night. I was sure everyone would notice my 117-pound loss tonight. The challenge was that the party was at Morton's of Chicago, home of very serious aged steaks. Most surgeons advise their patients to stay away from red meat for at least six months after surgery; it is often too difficult to digest. I really haven't missed it, but when we received the invitation, I started thinking about how good a few thin slices of filet mignon would taste.

Morton's is a very upscale steak house with dark wood paneling and a clubby feel to it, the kind of place with a cigar bar. Waiters fell over each other to keep a cocktail in your hand; huge silver platters of the biggest jumbo shrimp, absolutely enormous baked stuffed shrimp, tiny crab cakes, and baby lamb chops were carried around the room. The cocktail hour was not ending, and it looked like dinner was way off, so I decided to eat a shrimp and a crab cake. From 7:30 to 10:30 P.M. there was so much food I couldn't imagine how the rest of these folks were going to eat dinner. I drooled over the tiny lamb chops, but decided not to attempt that maneuver even though they looked very tender. One of our dear friends caught my eye from across the room and mouthed the words, "You look incredible, who are you?" Later on, when he made it across the room, he told me how perfect I looked. Then he backpedaled, and said that I was always beautiful but NOW! It is funny when people catch themselves gush-

ing over how great you look now but then don't want you to think
they thought that you were a slug before you lost the weight. It meant
a lot to me. I had been feeling a little fat—so many of the women were
emaciated.

We weren't seated for dinner until almost 11:00. We had our
choice of either a two-pound lobster out of the shell, a twenty-ounce
veal chop, or a double filet mignon. Ty ordered the lobster and I
ordered the filet but after an hour without the food appearing, I was
thinking that I should have eaten a few more shrimp. Not that I was
hungry, but I knew that I needed food. I was sipping some white wine
and it went straight to my head, slurring my speech within minutes.
It scared me and really freaked out my husband. He looked at me
and asked me if I was all right and grabbed my hand, but I couldn't
even answer him, my tongue was so thick. Then the feeling passed as
quickly as it had come over me and I felt a little dazed. They finally
put my food in front of me at almost midnight. The filet had to weigh
a pound! I sawed it in half and it was incredibly tender. This was an
utterly fabulous piece of meat. I had to really concentrate on chewing
it well. It actually made me a little sad that I could eat so little of it,
but I just didn't have the room. By this time it was after 12:30, and all
of us at the table were yawning while we ate. We decided to slip out
before dessert without making a fuss. I wish I had the rest of that filet
for tomorrow. Hell, I wish I had the rest of that filet to work on eating
for the whole next week!

April 5, 2002

It is a glorious day here at the beach! The ocean is aqua and smooth.
I am going to finish my protein shake and head out for a swim.
I made a cookies and cream shake this morning to try something
new and it tastes exactly like a Dairy Queen Blizzard. The key is
to use a half cup of skim milk or water, 2 scoops of a good vanilla

protein such as Isopure, and 1 cup of ice, and pulse the blender until the mixture is smooth and frosty. Then throw in two Murray's sugar-free chocolate cream-filled sandwich cookies and a tablespoon of Cool Whip and flip on the switch just long enough for the cookies to get sucked into the blades. It tastes amazing.

April 16, 2002

My grandmother will be 90 in May and my family has planned a party for her in New Jersey. This will be my first time on a plane since my surgery. Last night as I was choosing seats on the Expedia website, I had a flash of loathing for the middle seat and panicked about the flight. I never used a seat belt extender, as I would rather have died during a free fall in turbulence than face the humiliation of publicly requesting one. I would suck in to snap the seat belt, holding my breath until I passed the flight attendants' check, then quietly release the restraint without an audible click. I couldn't put my tray table down without it hitting my chest, so I had to say that I didn't want anything to eat or drink. Crowded flights were even more miserable, with my poor husband having to endure my being jammed into his side for hours so I didn't take up any of the window passenger's space. I can imagine how awful flying is for people who are even larger than I was. And of course, five out of ten times I would have a "recliner" in front of me. I would tap on the back of their seat, firmly telling them that with seats as close as they are on planes, there just wasn't enough room with their seat back, and could they please put it up. I know that even when I am thin, I will not recline on planes, knowing how uncomfortable it makes larger people who don't have the voice to say anything.

May 1, 2002

I am discovering that I can eat slightly larger quantities of food than I could initially, and that it would be easy to eat the wrong foods. I notice that some of the others who had their surgery about the same time as I did are really off track with the food choices they are making and the amount of sugar they know they can tolerate. My surgery was almost eleven months ago and I am not finished losing weight yet; I don't want to eat anything that will slow down my loss or prevent me from getting to my goal weight. There are women from my surgical support group who talk about eating at Taco Bell or Wendy's, and how much of a Subway sandwich they can consume. They laugh nervously about eating mini Snickers bars and how regular ice cream doesn't make them "dump." They eat baked potatoes, bread, rolls, and crackers, and think nothing of it because they are still limited in their volume. To me, every bite of carbohydrate prevents me from burning my stored fat. I have taken a completely different approach to using my pouch as a tool for life. I didn't enter into this process thinking that I would only have to change my diet for a few months and then could go back to eating the same way I did before my surgery. I made a resolution that I would change the way I made decisions about food and would make these changes permanent to my lifestyle. I just don't cook foods that don't work for my dietary requirements; I watch every gram of carbohydrate that I eat, and rarely buy bread or crackers anymore. There are times when I need something crunchy with my shrimp salad; but if I am going to eat a few crackers, I count them out and make sure that I compensate by having fewer carbohydrates for supper. I don't feel sad that I can't eat the entire box of Cheez-Its, I am thankful that I can eat ten of them while wearing size 12 jeans. Many people who have bariatric surgery don't realize that they have a seven- to ten-month window of opportunity to maximize their weight loss, and after that time the rate of loss declines drastically.

May 21, 2002

Grandma's birthday bash was wonderful and she never looked younger or more beautiful! I am so thankful for good genes, even if some of them are fat genes. Her skin is flawless, and her neck and chest aren't wrinkled at all. She is the epitome of classic Italian beauty—snow-white hair and sparkling hazel eyes with a touch of mischief in them—and still sharp as a razor and spry as a 40-year-old. When she realized that this was no ordinary birthday dinner she laughed, then cried tears of joy as she realized all her family had gathered to celebrate her 90 years of life. It was an incredible day and Grandma Helen proclaimed it the greatest day of her life. As she blew out the candles on her Italian cream cake she asked God for ten more years. I am sure he is working on it right now.

When she found out we were all taking her to Atlantic City in the morning, nothing else mattered for the evening. The next day we arrived to pick her up and she had prepared the Italian Grandma Special of manicotti, meatballs, and tossed salad. It was delicious and we all laughed as Grandma kept telling me to eat more food. When we arrived at the casino, Grandma practically ran through the lobby toward the slot machines, and walked up and down the aisles until she found the one she felt was ready to pay off. We knew where she would be for the next few hours, so we decided to find a blackjack table. I moved through the casino feeling great about myself, feeling light, feeling beautiful, feeling small, finally rid of the baggage I had carried for so many years. We played blackjack for six hours straight and our little pile of green chips grew to several piles of black chips— we were almost $3,000 ahead by suppertime. It was time to retrieve Grandma and the rest of the family, and since we were the big winners it would be our treat at the casino's gourmet seafood restaurant. How-ever, Grandma had beat us to it: she had gone to the host window and cashed in her "comps" to take all of us to dinner at the buffet. I couldn't eat the featured prime rib—it was too dense and dry—but she was so proud to take us all to dinner on her winnings that it didn't matter at all.

June 1, 2002

Just ten days to go to celebrate my one-year surgery date! I am leaving in two days on a trip to Germany with my brother, John. He works for Mercedes-Benz and one of his clients wanted a special-edition car that has a lengthy waiting list in the U.S. The only way for this man to get his hands on one of these cars is to take delivery in Europe under a special program. The Mercedes-Benz factory keeps a few of the really special cars such as the CL55 AMG for this select program, but this client really had no intention of going to Germany to get it. Yep, he plotted to send my brother, but didn't tell him until after he had ordered the car. So my brother has to pick up this incredible car from the factory in Stuttgart and enjoy the royal treatment that Mercedes-Benz lavishes on clients buying $115,000 cars. How do I fit into this picture? John's wife would never leave their three-year-old son, Alec, with anyone, not even to go to the store or the mall, and she surely wouldn't leave him for a week while she went to Germany with my brother. So, I told John that I would go with him! I fly out of Miami, he flies from Newark, we meet in London, then fly together to Stuttgart, Germany. I am so excited—I have never been to Europe before. My brother won't be driving the client's new car while we are in Germany; as much as he would love to take this mega-fast AMG car out on the Autobahn, a scratch would mean curtains for his job, so John will sign for it and take it to the parking lot on the other side of the factory, where it will be shipped to New Jersey. Then we rent our own smaller Benz and are off on our Black Forest rally. I didn't know anything about this area, but now that I have checked it out on the Internet, I know it is going to be fabulous. Of course I researched and found the name of the place that reportedly has the best Black Forest cake on the planet and learned how to say it in German even though I can only savor three bites of *Schwarzwälder Kirschtorte!* I told John to smack the fork from my hand if I go for a fourth bite or he would be carrying me out of the place. The area is also known for its handmade sausages and cured hams. I am packing plenty of protein bars and two packs of ready-to-drink protein shakes just in case I can't eat.

I decided that on the way home, instead of just changing planes at Heathrow, I would stay a night in London to celebrate my one-year anniversary date. My brother has to continue on home, but being alone is not a bad thing. I am celebrating my newfound strength and life. While I would love to be with my husband, this time alone is not so bad. I am going to check into the Connaught, one of London's finest hotels. I can't wait to go to dinner at the finest restaurant in London and raise my glass in a toast "to Susan." I am pissed that Paul McCartney is getting married this week. I am a week too late to win the heart of my favorite Beatle. Celebrating my one-year birthday at 149 pounds in London is going to be the best part. I will drink in all the flavors and take in the sights and have a great trip. Life just gets better and better all the time as I get smaller and smaller! Paul's loss.

June 11, 2002

One year ago yesterday I began my new life. I cannot believe this past year and how much has changed for me. I returned from the most fabulous trip of my life late last night and none of it would have happened without my surgery last June.

I am 147 pounds this morning, so I have lost 131 pounds in this very full and remarkable year. I should be winding down with losing but I am sure that I will continue to slowly lose over the next few months, which is fine with me. The size-10 BCBG jeans I bought for my trip were a little big yesterday so I am sure eights are coming by next month. I dwell on how I look sometimes because it is amazing to look in the mirror and see someone you don't recognize as you, but I walked for miles around Germany and London with extra energy and climbed mountains of stairs and could have gone on forever. That is what this procedure is all about: health and fitness. The fact that I regained lost beauty and youth is a gift!

Germany was incredible; the country is simply the most beautiful place I have ever been. Picking up John's client's car was a blast; we had a tour of the Mercedes-Benz factory and were treated to a gourmet dinner in their elegant restaurant. White asparagus are in peak season at the moment, and all the restaurants in this area celebrate the greatly anticipated, short season by having a *Spargelkart*, or asparagus menu, with four- and five-course dinners that feature these delicate rarities. So my "foodie" brother and I dove right in and had cream of asparagus soup, asparagus salad, and asparagus with hollandaise and prawns as the main course, a large pile of tender logs of white asparagus napped with the delicious classic lemon butter sauce. The prawns were there as an afterthought, as the asparagus were the centerpiece of this amazing dish. I had never tasted fresh white asparagus before but they were incredible with a very delicate flavor. I sliced the thick spears into thin slices and with the sauce had no trouble eating about half of my pile of ten spears.

The hotels that Mercedes-Benz chooses for the Euro delivery clients are amazing. To say that the Schlosshotel Bühlerhöhe was luxurious is an understatement. A grand hotel and spa built at the turn of the twentieth century, it has been completely and magnificently restored. The views are breathtaking, taking in miles of mountains with the Swiss Alps in the distance. We were treated like royalty with an international array of polite and crisp waiters and butlers catering to our every whim. A wonderful European custom is to have a late afternoon snack of tea or coffee and pastry. We had caffé macchiatos and I selected a rhubarb cream torte from the pastry cart. It had a buttery shortbread crust, with a thick layer of tangy buttermilk or yogurt custard topped with tart sliced rhubarb; not a sweet pastry by any means, but as it was definitely not sugar-free I gathered up all my willpower and ate a little of the large slice, not wanting to test my dumping mechanism in the middle of this grand drawing room. It was heavenly and I found that I have a very good handle on my willpower when it is backed by fear. My brother had his first of many large hunks of Black Forest cake—German chocolate cake layered with whipped cream and cherries soaked in the local cherry liqueur. The bite I sampled was ethereal.

We spent the afternoon exploring the area and had a late dinner in our hotel's celebrated restaurant. The rain had started to fall and our views were now of the milky white clouds that obscured our earlier panorama. Dinner was fabulous but my brother still could not get over the fact that I never eat more than half of what's on my plate. He did comment though that I was not a cheap date, since I still order the same plate of food; I am a *wasteful* date. I ordered a coffee crème brûlée for dessert; it was silky and cold with the hot crisp caramelized sugar crust on top, served with a plate of fresh plum compote and a platter of petits fours that were miniature works of art! John didn't want dessert but once this extravagance was put in front of me and I only ate three spoonfuls of the crème brûlée, he picked up the spoon and finished off all the sweet treats, mumbling what a waste it would be to not eat this incredible food.

After one year, dumping syndrome is still a very real fear to me. I have not tested my limits; in fact I am careful not to cross my self-imposed line of 5 to 8 grams of sugar at one time. I don't feel deprived, rather I feel blessed that I can enjoy a formal or gourmet meal including an incredible dessert and stay within my boundaries of carbohydrates and sugar. This surgical procedure has given me strength, and is a tool that allows me to taste but not overeat. I have friends who have tested their sugar limits and are distraught that they do not dump, thereby giving them permission to step out of the RNY limits and cheat. I am convinced that these folks will regain some of their weight and have a harder time maintaining long-term weight loss even with the surgical limitations of their stomach volume. I have to be satisfied with a taste of dessert backed with the fear of dumping. Later that night, I kept repeating this to myself in order to keep my hand from stuffing the handmade chocolates that I found on my nightstand directly into my mouth.

Our flight touched down in London and I tearfully said good-bye to my wonderful brother at Heathrow airport. John and I have cooked together and talked food for years and there is no one I know of in this world who could have been as perfectly paired with him to share this epicurean journey. I grabbed the London express train and within a half hour of landing at Heathrow was sitting by myself in the magnificent lobby of my London hotel. The Connaught is old money, old world, old attitude, and incredibly stuffy; I loved it. Would Madame like a pot of tea while the bellman takes her bags up to her room and her butler unpacks for her? Absolutely! I thought of my mother and I knew she was watching over me and smiling while I enjoyed my moment of extreme sophistication.

I finished my tea, then climbed the staircase up to my room, where my mind was immediately blown! The room was just lovely, with fabrics in bright yellows, greens, and touches of burgundy, a Louis XIV writing desk, a goose down comforter and linen duvet, eight linen-covered down pillows piled against the headboard, a magnificent green Murano glass chandelier hanging from the ceiling, a massive antique mahogany wardrobe, a thick Frette terry robe to luxuriate in, and a marble bath with shining silver fixtures. I changed my clothes and headed out to explore London.

I am writing all this in such detail because just a year ago I would have never done any of it! I wouldn't have had the guts to get on a plane and head off to Germany, never mind be in London by myself. As a fat girl I was too self-conscious, always thinking people were looking at me and judging me, laughing at me. Maybe they were, and maybe they weren't, but it sure stopped me from living. The new me is free and bold, as I love life and myself. So don't think that I am getting too far off topic. While in London I feel tall, I feel thin, and I feel beautiful.

I bought a ticket and boarded a double-decker bus. I was the only patron and as I climbed the narrow metal spiral staircase to the top deck the reality struck me that not too many months ago I was too large to fit. Perched high atop the moving bus, I had a wonderful vantage point for all of London's sights and a personal tour guide to explain everything I was seeing. I had a great afternoon with James, my tour guide, even when the inevitable London rain commenced. After the tour, I said good-bye to James and my bus driver and walked back to the hotel with my mascara streaming down my face, looking a bit like Ozzie Osbourne, my hair in soaked ringlets around my face. I was miserably wet. The doorman recognized my pitiful condition and suggested that I have some hot tea in the drawing room. That sounded good to me. I sat down and in minutes the formal white-gloved waiter placed a silver tea service in front of me. There were six kinds of sugar—brown rock crystals, white rock crystals, brown cubes, white cubes, brown granules, white granules—but just one kind of sugar substitute: an envelope with two tiny white saccharin pills. I drank my tea plain, with just a touch of cream, rather than taint it with saccharin. The concierge came over and asked me if Madame would like him to have my butler draw me a hot bath while Madame drank her tea. After her tea, Madame had a hot bath and when she was finished the sun was shining, so Madame dried off, did her makeup and hair, got dressed, this time grabbing an umbrella from the concierge, and was off on round two of her adventure! Walk, walk, walk, walk, walk, walk, walk, walk, walk, walk, walk, walk—wow, what energy I have at 147 pounds!

The 300-pound Susan would have stayed in the hotel—actually the 300-pound Susan would be sitting at home in Florida. I had a bounce in my step and all the confidence in the world as I made my way around this gorgeous city.

When I glanced at my watch, I couldn't believe how quickly time had passed and that it was time for the appointment I had made for the London Eye. The British Airways Millennium Wheel is a 50-story, constantly moving observation wheel with 25 giant glass pods that allow amazing views over the city of London and the countryside. I quickly located it in the skyline and ran so I wouldn't miss my reservation. I was upset that I had arrived ten minutes after my time slot. But when I swiped my Visa in the machine to retrieve my ticket, out popped the ticket. I stood on the platform and thought about times I had dreaded stepping onto an elevator because of the embarrassing lurch my weight would cause—and here I was ready to step into a huge glass egg without hesitation. A beautiful family from India and a local London family who pointed out the sites were my mates for this trip as we ascended to almost 500 feet in the sky. What an incredible feeling of freedom. It was almost 9:00 P.M. yet the stone buildings of London were reflecting the glow of the bright orange late-afternoon sun as we slowly rotated around the giant spoked wheel. It was simply breathtaking.

The Connaught has a Michelin-starred restaurant, and since I was alone, I thought it best to eat in the hotel rather than wander London after dark. I dashed upstairs and fluffed my hair, jazzed up my makeup, stopped for a minute to celebrate the fact that I could now wear size B pantyhose, slipped on a slinky black T dress, slid into my high heels, wrapped my new French blue cashmere pashmina around my shoulders, and added blue topaz and diamond earrings and bracelets. I felt like Princess Diana as I descended the stairs to the lobby. The maître d' welcomed me, seated me facing the room at a lovely table, and I suddenly had all eyes of the room upon me.

I sipped my Kir Royale—champagne with just a drop of Chambord liqueur—and softly smiled while I studied the menu for easy-to-eat choices in one of the world's finest restaurants. I decided on the terrine of foie gras as an appetizer and the roasted Dover sole served with an English mustard-butter sauce and sautéed baby spinach. The terrine was incredible, but I ate just half of the thin slice knowing that room in my pouch was limited. I ignored the bread basket on my table, though with great difficulty. The Dover sole was presented in an enormous silver domed platter and set atop a silver frame while the waiter expertly deboned the whole roasted fish and plated it, spooning on the creamy mustard sauce. I ate about half of the moist, perfectly cooked and seasoned fish along with a few bites of the sautéed spinach before I became very full. I sipped a crisp Chardonnay along with my fish, selected by the sommelier to go with my sole. I never drink with my meals but this was the exception. The waiters fell over themselves to take care of me and keep me entertained. After my meal, the headwaiter tempted me with the dessert cart and after I explained I had to choose a less-sugared dessert because I was a "diabetic," we discussed the merits of each of the desserts on the cart. He could have the dessert chef prepare a simple compote of stewed, unsweetened fresh fruits as there were bowls of poached apricots, pitted cherries, strawberries, rhubarb, and pears; or I could choose a decadent and fabulous sugary creation knowing I couldn't risk a fourth bite. John had convinced me that a tiny taste of something spectacular was better than a whole lot of something ordinary. I chose a Spring Cup, a beautifully etched martini glass holding thin, even layers of pistachio mousse, dense, tart apricot puree, bittersweet chocolate mousse, milk chocolate mousse, and vanilla-bean cream. The colors in this dessert were so soft and beautiful that if its stripes were of silk it would be my favorite scarf. It was a work of art and I precisely measured out a reasonable amount of this unreasonable dessert on my spoon and slowly let it dissolve in my mouth. The flavors were incredible and intense.

After savoring a safe amount, I pushed the plate to the far side of the table and it was quickly whisked away. I smiled as I climbed the winding dark wood staircase to my room. The butler had turned down my bed and the fine linens felt so soft and wonderful. I thought about my spectacular day in London and fell into a deep sleep. For the first time in many years I was confident that there was no way that my dreams could possibly surpass the reality of this past week.

July 22, 2002

My husband and I were having dinner at the Fifth Avenue Grill on Friday evening, a celebration dinner of sorts for a couple of big deals we closed earlier that day, when I casually suggested that we should go to Las Vegas this weekend. Or maybe it was my husband who said it first, I really don't recall. Maybe it was his Beefeater martini or possibly my Peppar Bloody Mary that made it seem like a great suggestion, but we both jumped on it. When we got home I logged onto Orbitz.com, found two nonstop tickets to Las Vegas, threw a few things in our bags, and we headed to the airport. A tuxedoed driver in his silver limousine met us, compliments of the Mirage, and within six hours of our dinner, we were checking in at the VIP office of one of the most exciting places in the world.

It was 2:00 A.M. Las Vegas time, and the Mirage was as beautiful as I remembered. We took the private elevator to our floor, quickly unpacked, regrouped, and were at a blackjack table in 20 minutes, playing cards and having a ball until dawn. We staggered upstairs and got a couple of hours sleep courtesy of the room-darkening shades before my ultimate bariatric test: the Mirage brunch buffet. I used to dream about this buffet; my husband used to tease me about having prime rib for breakfast in my old life. I was hesitant about standing in front of the largest food orgy in Las Vegas and trying to select a few bites of protein, but I was up for the challenge. Was the quality as good as the quantity or was the sheer volume what I had loved about this buffet in the past? I grabbed a large plate and decided on some chilled jumbo shrimp, a cheese blintz, and a few slices of smoked salmon to roll up with cream cheese, red onion, and capers. It was hard not to let my eyes be too much bigger than my stomach. It is tough to take one of something small, but I am learning. Everything was delicious and I didn't miss the mountains of food on my plate at all. Sitting there in size-10 jeans was no doubt a factor. Food no longer rules me, but I still went back to the dessert buffet and got a tiny espresso cup of crème brûlée to satisfy my love for the stuff and had my obligatory spoonful. I was stuffed and overjoyed.

Back at the blackjack tables, we spent hours attempting to break the house. All day long we were up and down, never quite reaching my husband's goal in order to quit winners. We had a blast and laughed as we had twenty years ago when he first took me to Las Vegas.

During a break from the tables we strolled past the jewelry shop to look at watches and I spied a gorgeous David Yurman ring that matched a bracelet I had bought there with blackjack winnings eight years ago. I have lost so much weight that all my rings fall off my fingers and seem too large in style for my now more petite hands. Even my diamond wedding band needs to be completely remade, as the thick, size 10½ pavé band is ridiculously large. The ring in the case was a gorgeous gold and silver twisted band featuring a large, faceted peridot stone. I left the store with the ring and the matching earrings. Life is cool.

The next 24 hours were a blur of blackjack, a romantic lobster tail dinner in the middle of the Mirage rainforest, a great show, and more blackjack. We caught our limo at the north entrance of the hotel and were deposited at the airport at 11:00 P.M. for our red-eye flight home to Miami. We walked in the door of our condo at 9:00 A.M. yesterday morning and I sit here laughing about our whirlwind blackjack tour of the Mirage. Only the dazzling ring on my finger confirms our last two days of spontaneity and laughter!

September 2, 2002

I celebrated my forty-first birthday on August 30th. I wasn't upset about it, though. I was upset on my fortieth birthday because I was so huge and joked at the time that forty-one and thin would be much better than forty and fat. It is true! Being forty-one years old is extraordinary. We celebrated with dinner at Morton's, and I wore the magnificent blouse I bought at a boutique in the Mirage Shops in Vegas. It is all leopard and lace print in browns, black, and white, shredded, crinkled, and see-through; it wraps around my body and ties, showing major cleavage, and the sleeves are long and uneven. It is so cool and sexy; I love it! Ty looked pretty good too—he is a striking man and we really look good together again. I had a Peppar Bloody Mary and he had a Beefeater martini, along with some tiny West Coast oysters, of which I ate two. I ordered filet Oscar, a seared filet mignon, butterflied and topped with lump crabmeat and perfect hollandaise sauce. Ty, being a fish-eating vegetarian, ordered crab cakes. The filet was fork tender; I ate almost one half of the moist, crab-topped steak before I was very full. We lingered and the waiter brought over the dessert tray. We decided on cappuccino and I chose the cheesecake. My husband wanted me to choose Key lime pie. I told him that it had too much sugar and that I wanted a bite of cheesecake. He made a face and said he wanted me to get the pie, as in his opinion Key lime pie is better than cheesecake. I pulled rank and firmly told him that he didn't get to choose, since it is *my* birthday! So I had now inadvertently informed the waiter that it was my birthday. Thanks a lot, Ty; now I had candles on my cheesecake as it crossed the room. But at least the waiters didn't sing to me. The upshot was that I won and got a bite of cheesecake, plus it was on the house. It was a fun evening and we strolled hand in hand from the restaurant even after the ugly cheese-cake incident.

September 12, 2002

It is miraculous how even the way you think about food changes during the months after your surgery. Now that I am fifteen months post-op I suddenly feel so normal about eating small portions. I really enjoy good food even with a stomach the size of a small lemon. I savor the food and take pleasure in the flavors. I eat slowly, actually putting my fork down while chewing and tasting, instead of finishing my entire plate in minutes. When I look at the menu I select something that appeals to me rather than thinking about the portion size. I don't worry that the crab appetizer I order for my entrée will be small. I weigh the value of each morsel and prioritize what I want to put into my mouth, eating the best bites first. I think about what I really want and what will work for me; it isn't a mindless overindulgence anymore. I cannot believe how my entire relationship with food has changed.

My sudden weight loss has left me with an unsightly flap of skin hanging from my lower belly called a panniculus. The surgical procedure in which this skin is removed, called a panniculectomy, is usually performed in tandem with a tightening of the underlying abdominal muscles, or abdominoplasty. I had a consultation with a plastic surgeon on Tuesday and scheduled my reconstructive surgery. I really like the no-nonsense approach of the surgeon, and the fact that he was a professor at Duke University Medical School. Dr. Rainer Sachse performed a hernia operation, surgical scar revision, and tummy tuck on my girlfriend Dhona; her scar is amazingly thin and well hidden, and her stomach is completely flat and taut. He was very confident that he could remove all of the excess belly fat and skin from my stomach using a slightly extended version of the regular abdominoplasty scar going about six inches past each of my hipbones. I am very fortunate that my arms and legs are small, with little excess skin; all my extra weight is in my lower stomach. I can actually grab it with my hands and pull it away from my abdomen, similar to what the surgeon will be doing with this operation. I will be so small when those 8 pounds of fat and skin are gone. It is frightening to me to go under general anesthesia again, but I cannot imagine going through all this and not completing the last few yards. I don't think that I need the abdominoplasty procedure but I do want it. The date is set for October 24, 2002. All the surgeons I interviewed said that there is no way insurance will cover a dime of the procedure because my skin flap doesn't even lap over, so I will have to pay for it myself.

I have been going through the emotions of my gastric bypass surgery again as my girlfriend Jo had her laparoscopic RNY surgery last Thursday; she is one week post-op today and is doing absolutely fantastically. She spent just two nights in the hospital and was feeling pretty funky the first night, but after that there was no stopping her from walking up and down those halls. Her surgeon is a little different with his initial food requirements in that she is to stick to clear liquids for an additional week, so I made a pot of homemade chicken broth today to take to her house in the morning. When I was one week post-op I was still sitting in my hospital bed sucking on ice chips, but when I returned home I really appreciated a steaming mug of homemade chicken broth—it was so soothing and warm going down. Jo is 66, a retired special education teacher who lives next door to my dad. She watched in awe as I melted before her eyes over the past year. She shocked all of us when she announced that she was going to have the surgery. Many of her friends tried to talk her out of it, telling her she was too old. She weighed the positives and negatives and made her decision based on the facts as they pertained to her. Jo decided that she was 66 years young, not old, and that she was heading down a rough road weighing 235 pounds at a mere

4 feet, 10 inches. She is already telling the naysayers that "nothing tastes as good as thin feels" when they ask her if she misses eating. She is a good student and she is going to be so cute when she is little. She reminds me quite frequently that she is the same height as Judy Garland, and is such a great lady. Her blood pressure has already dropped to normal levels, her cholesterol has plummeted, and she is full of energy.

October 5, 2002

We went on the annual Harley-Davidson Key West Poker Run with some of our yuppie biker friends. What fun! You leave Miami and while en route to Key West you make five designated stops, choosing a playing card from a deck of cards at each stop. At the last stop the person with the best poker hand wins either cash or a new Harley. There were over 10,000 motorcycles participating, even with Hurricane Isadore swirling in the gulf. From the back of the V-Rod I enjoyed the perfect vantage point to watch hundreds of motorcycles cruising over the seven-mile bridge in Marathon Key with the turquoise water, and palm trees swaying in the background. Life was a postcard! Downtown was packed and I got to be a bad biker mama for the weekend. Two of the wives asked me why I didn't just let go and splurge for a special occasion. They had noticed how careful I am about what I eat. I just reiterated that I didn't like to be overstuffed when I was on the motorcycle and left it at that. I feel guilty that they admire my control. If they only knew.

When we got home I discovered that my friend Jo had been hospitalized! Apparently she didn't think that water was important and she wasn't drinking any. She also wasn't eating enough food and didn't want to drink the protein shakes I told her she should be sipping. She was taken to the emergency room while we were in Key West and they admitted her and gave her two IVs for severe dehydration. So with Ty in bed at home, sick with bronchitis, I left him to go to the hospital every day because Jo was a total wreck, crying and whimpering. She was scared to death she was dying. I needed to hold her hand and keep telling her that she didn't have anything wrong with her that would kill her, but if she didn't start drinking water, I would kill her. After eleven days, she is home and has learned that food and water are important after weight-loss surgery. If you are having a problem that prevents you from eating or drinking, you have to call your surgeon's office. Jo cannot cook to save her life, so once I took her home I went to the store and bought some cooked shrimp, turkey breast, cheese, cottage cheese, and canned premixed chocolate protein shakes. I chopped the cooked shrimp and blended them with a couple of spoonfuls of low-sugar cocktail sauce so it would be moist, and put the bowl in her refrigerator. I cooked some sugar-free chocolate pudding and whisked in a couple of scoops of protein powder. I instructed her to eat little portions, to make sure she waits an hour after eating before drinking, and to sip water constantly while walking. This time she is going to be fine. I am not sure she knew that it wasn't all cake and roses from 278 pounds to where I am now. It takes dedication to health, and you must follow the rules of eating and, just as important, drinking. Sixty-four ounces of water doesn't seem like a lot until you are on your third eight-ounce glass of the day, which you are managing to funnel through a very small opening.

October 22, 2002

While we were on a weekend trip to Daytona Beach on our Harley, we decided to head over to Universal Studios in Orlando for the day. We had a light breakfast and were pulling through the Universal Studio's gates in about an hour. We practically ran through the gates of Islands of Adventures and stopped short to gaze at the incredible roller coasters. I hadn't been on a ride in years. I would never admit that it was because of my weight, but now I am certain that I was afraid of not fitting on the rides. I know people who had to face the humiliation of not being able to fit in the seat, or being too large for the restraint device to lock. I stared at the Incredible Hulk roller coaster and had to try it. As the hydraulic bar locked into place over my body, I was secretly relieved that it fit. It was an irrational fear but my heart still raced. I started screaming from the moment I was first turned upside-down and didn't stop until my feet were back on the ground. I can't believe I had convinced myself I didn't like this kind of ride. On to Fire and Ice Dueling Dragons, two separate roller coasters that intertwine; when you are on Fire, your body is flying mere inches away from the people who are riding on Ice. We decided to have a snack as Ty spied a candy shop. There were huge bins of sugar-free Jelly Belly jelly beans in delicious flavors and I filled a bag with almost a pound of the intensely fruity candies. I placed the open bag in my leather Harley pouch and started munching on them as we walked through the rest of the park. While we were considering our next roller coaster ride I felt the unmistakable rumble of my stomach telling me that I was getting ready to have an immediate and severe problem. I had eaten almost half of the sugar-free candy, which doesn't affect blood sugar levels because maltitol sweetener isn't absorbed in the intestines. However, there are warnings on foods containing maltitol and I was about to have a lesson confirming why this is so. It was very stupid to eat that much sugar-free candy, and after a brief restroom tour of the park, I was ready to leave.

October 27, 2002

It is less than three days since I went in for my plastic surgery procedure and I feel terrific! I have felt wonderful since the moment I opened my eyes after my surgery. I never experienced that horrible, groggy, heavy headache feeling from the anesthesia. This anesthesiologist must have done something different. I felt awful when I woke up from my other two surgeries, but this one was like waking up from a nap. I had no pain to speak of, just a fear of moving! I started to get a bit nauseous and the nurse put an alcohol pad to my nose and the feeling went away immediately. Nice trick. They helped me up from the bed and walked me over to a recliner chair. I put on my sweatpants and zippered sweatshirt and felt great. I was moving slowly but it was from the thick bandages and drains hanging from the bandages. I cannot stand up straight and have to walk hunched over. I decided that my own bed would be a wonderful thing and soon I was in a wheelchair heading toward my car. My sweet husband had brought a pillow for me to hug, but I really didn't need it. I was alert but a little foggy now and then. I don't remember the trip, but I did get nauseous in our elevator and had to spit up just as I was walking to my bedroom. Poor Ty was walking with all my stuff and didn't know what I needed, and of course my mouth was full of spit. I just stood there looking at the little pink dish he was holding. I finally snatched it from him and then remembered that I had an alcohol pad in my pocket that the nurse gave me just in case. It worked in time and I didn't throw up. Minor tragedy averted, as I am sure that throwing up would have hurt. Ty fixed my pillows so that I could sit up against the headboard. He had at least eight pillows for me, and propped up my legs and arms so I was comfy. I dozed off for a few hours but then woke with great clarity and can honestly say that I felt so much better than I had anticipated. I took several naps and started on my pain pills and antibiotics, making sure I ate a cracker with each pill to avoid nausea.

When I am in bed and look down at myself, it is like gazing at someone else's body. I don't recognize my own torso; it looks nothing like anything I have seen for the past 40 years. When the bandages are removed, I have a nice new deep belly button and a wide expanse of flat belly, and my abdomen flows neatly into my narrow hips. Granted, I look as if I have been nearly severed in half, but I'm not all bruised and swollen as I thought I would be. This is simply amazing. On June 10, 2001, I was 278 pounds and miserable, and this morning, except for the stitches, I am happy and look like I could be in a magazine. A shower can only improve things.

November 4, 2002

This is Day 11 post-op abdominoplasty and my drains are still in. Once I get them out I will be 100 percent back to normal within a day or two. I am sure that my body is fighting the intrusion of the couple of feet of plastic tubing, draining me of energy. I have been out of the house a couple of times but I am just too worried that I will rip out a tube by catching it on something, so my excursions have been limited. The incision is perfect except for a one-inch segment that looks a bit rough. I have only a few very faint bruises and my new belly button is a very attractive, vertically oriented little oval! My stitches are on the inside, no staples or black thread, just a perfectly, smoothly matched incision where the skin comes together. I have some swelling but already I have a nice smooth line now that I have switched to a high-waisted elastic panty garment. This surgery has gone perfectly for me. My friend Stephanie has had her tummy tuck as well. Her surgeon was apparently too aggressive and may have removed too much tissue and stretched her skin too tightly, compromising the blood supply between her new belly button and incision. This is called *tissue necrosis* and I don't think that she understands that she is going to have a lengthy recovery. I do believe that her wound is going to get much worse before it gets better, and this will be incredibly traumatic for her. Once again I am incredibly thankful for my excellent surgeon.

November 19, 2002

I am now four weeks post-op abdominoplasty and I feel fantastic! Drains are out, the incision is a faint pink line, and I have very little swelling remaining. I have a perfectly flat stomach! I can finally fit into my pre-op clothes, and they are big in the area below the waistband. They fit in the waist but there is this big baggy area where I used to have all the belly flab. I stare at myself in the mirror all the time; I can't believe that I am this thin. Now that the swelling has subsided, I can wear any size eight and actually fit into some size six skirts and pants. My mind is totally blown! When I had the weight-loss surgery I set my goal conservatively at a size 12 and decided that if I didn't get any smaller than that I would still be thrilled. I can't even imagine wearing a size six. I don't feel that small and in fact I still judge the spaces where I need to walk. I thought about it the other day when I got up from a restaurant table and went around the long way to avoid having to squeeze between chairs even though there was plenty of room. I was making my calculations based on the 278-pound body size instead of my new smaller mass. I wonder if I will ever feel small without looking in a mirror.

For the first time since having my weight-loss surgery, I experienced "dumping syndrome" from too much sugar while I was visiting Ty's family in Georgia. I have been so careful to avoid it over the past eighteen months. We were celebrating Uncle Billy's birthday at the farm and his daughter Barbara had baked a cake for him. I ate one layer of a thin slice of the cake, somehow completely misjudging the sugar grams that I was ingesting. Within minutes, I began to sweat profusely and got very dizzy. I asked Ty to take me outside so I could walk around in the cold fresh air, but then I had to come right back in and sit down on the sofa. I was hoping to avoid a scene and just stay in the living room while everyone finished their dessert. Then my stomach and intestines started to seize up inside of me and I had horrible abdominal pain. I thought I was going to die and unfortunately all of my in-laws thought so, too. Everyone gathered around me and kept asking me if I was all right. I was in absolute agony for about twenty minutes and didn't move for lack of knowing what the hell I was going to do. When I would breathe I would feel a sharp, stabbing pain in the area of my stomach pouch and intestines so I took shallow gulps of air. Then as fast as it came over me, it subsided and I was perfectly fine. I will be so much more careful from now on. I knew I shouldn't have had that last bite or two of cake. I am very upset that I did this to my-self, but now I know that I have to be careful to avoid sugar for the rest of my life. I don't ever want to experience dumping syndrome again!

I am healed from my surgeries in a physical sense, but this dump-ing episode proves to me that I will always have to be aware of my weight-loss surgery. I can be normal and run with the pack, but I can never forget the extreme measures I have gone through to get to where I am right now.

questions and answers about weight-loss surgery

These are the questions that I had and that people ask most frequently on websites.

What are the different kinds of weight-loss surgery, and which is the best?

There are primarily two restrictive procedures that are widely available in the United States for the surgical control of weight loss: gastric bypass (RNY), laparoscopic adjustable gastric band (Lap-Band), and gastric sleeve.

The gastric bypass, Roux-en-Y procedure is considered at this time to be the gold standard of bariatric surgery. This procedure reduces the stomach to a small pouch with a capacity to hold only a minimal amount of food, and bypasses a portion of the small intestine to add a mild malabsorptive element, meaning that not even all of the small amount of food eaten can be fully absorbed. Weight loss of 80 to 100 percent of excess body weight is readily achievable for most patients, and long-term maintenance of weight loss has proven to be extremely successful. This procedure provides a very good balance of weight loss, metabolic side effects, and surgical risk.

The laparoscopic adjustable gastric band procedure offers another way to limit food intake by placing a silicon band completely around the top end of the stomach. Surgical placement of the band is done laparoscopically; the device is lined with an inflatable balloon, allowing the surgeon to adjust the size of the band and rate of weight loss by adding or removing fluid from a reservoir that is just under the skin. Since the digestive process remains intact, patients must comply with a strict post-op diet and exercise regimen to achieve and maintain results.

Implantation of a Lap-Band device is a less invasive procedure that does not carry either the surgical risks or nutritional and mineral deficiencies of other bariatric procedures.

The rate of weight loss with the laparoscopic adjustable gastric band is slower than that with the gastric bypass, with patients maintaining an average of 54 percent of their weight loss at five years. Complications of the adjustable band include port problems, band erosions and slippage, or failure to lose a significant amount of weight.

The gastric sleeve is promoted as simple, but surgical removal of 80 percent of the stomach is disconcerting.

Only through careful research and discussion with qualified bariatric surgeons can you decide which procedure might be the best for your particular medical situation.

How do I know that my insurance will cover this procedure?

Surgical treatment of morbid obesity is medically necessary because it is the only proven method of achieving long-term weight control. Select a qualified bariatric surgeon, and after your consultation, the individual in their office who works directly with the insurance providers will issue a letter of medical necessity to your medical insurance carrier to authorize the procedure. Many times this specialized person in the surgeon's office deals with a specific person at each insurance company and can get an answer in a few days regarding your approval.

It generally appears that the larger centers performing more surgeries have better track records in securing insurance authorizations, since they are better tuned in to the details of what each insurance carrier requires for approval. There are so many kinds of insurance and so many different versions of each policy that it is difficult to accurately address insurance coverage issues even in general terms.

Now that I have decided to have gastric bypass surgery I can't seem to stop eating. Does everyone look at each meal as a last meal opportunity?

Once I had my date for surgery, every meal was my last meal. I packed on a good 10 to 15 pounds just prior to my surgery, thinking that I would never be able to eat again after my weight-loss surgery.

Once you have reached your weight goal there really isn't anything that you can't have at least a bite or two of. Just before surgery, I ate huge steaks with fully loaded baked potatoes, piles of fried shrimp, five or six large slices of pizza in a sitting, hunks of cheesecake—and it was all so silly in retrospect. Now that I am at my goal weight, I eat steak, savor a few bites of potato, practically live on shrimp, and occasionally have the toppings from a small slice of pizza or sugar-free cheesecake, if I choose. I can have a bite or two of anything that I want; my small stomach pouch gives me the control, and I am completely satisfied with just a taste. So my advice is to have a pint of Ben & Jerry's Chubby Hubby, and go to a decadent Sunday brunch buffet at a fancy hotel and get your money's worth for the last time . . . but remember that once you are at your goal weight you can have a little of anything you choose.

What items are important for me to take to the hospital?
I overpacked for my hospital stay and never even opened my small
suitcase. Forget the nightgowns, toiletries, and makeup; if you are
feeling good enough to care how you look, they will send you home
in five minutes. The things that I appreciated and would recommend are:

- Baby wipes. It is very difficult to wash your hands properly
  with an IV in your forearm or hand. After taking a few laps
  while pushing your IV pole, touching doorknobs, or being
  transported via wheelchair for testing, it is good to be able to
  clean your hands. It feels good to be able to wash your face
  and sponge bathe in bed.
- A small squeeze bottle and liquid body soap. If your size causes
  you to have some difficulty with personal bathroom hygiene, it
  becomes even more difficult immediately after your surgery or
  even impossible depending on your IV placement. For some,
  using the moistened baby wipes will be sufficient. You can also
  fill your squeeze bottle with warm, soapy water and use it to rinse
  yourself while sitting on the commode. Dry yourself by sitting on
  a clean towel that you have placed on the side of your hospital
  bed. In the hospital these squeeze bottles are called "episiotomy
  bottles" and are commonly used on the maternity floors.
- Women should have a supply of maxi pads: surgery frequently
  causes a sudden onset of menstrual bleeding, even if not
  expected, and since we are given blood thinners, it can be
  unusually heavy.
- Something comfortable to wear home. You will probably have
  a drain protruding from your abdomen, and even with a
  laparoscopic procedure you won't want anything resting on
  your incisions. You may also be larger than when you checked

into the hospital because of bloat and swelling. Pack a pair of sweatpants or leggings with a soft wide waistband to wear rolled below your belly, and a long loose T-shirt that hides everything, along with slip-on shoes.

- Lip balm. Your lips will be very crusty and dry after your procedure, and you may not receive a cup of ice chips for some time. Lip balm is priceless in this instance.

- A favorite pillow. It will be difficult to get comfortable in your hospital bed. Having the perfect pillow from your own bed is very reassuring. Press it into your stomach when you have to get out of bed, and hug it to your belly during the car ride home to cushion the impact of road bumps.

Exactly what kind of pain will I experience for the first few days?

When I woke up I wasn't in pain, I just felt incredibly foggy and absolutely terrible. I had nausea and an overall feeling of confusion. I couldn't concentrate on anything anyone said to me, and would fall in and out of consciousness. I wasn't taken back to my room until late in the evening because I was my surgeon's last patient, so the nurses gave me a brief reprieve and allowed me to sleep. My girlfriend Ronni slept in the next bed and I did have to wake her up in the middle of the night so that she could help me use the bathroom. The nurse moved my bed into a sitting position and pulled my legs around so I found myself sitting on the edge of my bed with my feet on the floor. I held a pillow against my abdomen as I stood up. The pain was not debilitating—I rated it a six out of ten. First thing in the morning the nurse helped me out of bed and had me walking around the central nurses' station. I was still very groggy and although I wasn't in much pain, I did have a very hard time staying awake as I walked. My surgeon uses injections and then oral medications for pain management and does not use the pain pumps that some surgeons prefer.

Many of us describe the way we feel during the first post-op days in terms of the size of the truck that hit us, but we are talking about an overall dreadful feeling and not one of great pain. This seems to hold true in cases of both laparoscopic and open procedures.

I am four weeks post-op laparoscopic RNY surgery and I have a pain in my left side. When will it go away?

The reason your left side hurts is because it is through these openings that most of the laparoscopic action takes place. These are the holes that the larger instruments are manipulated through, so there is more injury to your tissue in this area. It is normal for these sites to cause some discomfort for a few weeks. In order to give them time to heal, it is important that you not do any lifting or bending while you have this pain; no emptying the dishwasher or the dryer, or picking up the cat dishes from the floor. If you don't already have standing approval from your doctor to take Tylenol, give him a call and follow his recommendation for pain control.

Will I need plastic surgery?

Not everyone desires or even needs reconstructive plastic surgery after the large weight loss following gastric bypass surgery. Factors such as age, your starting weight, and where you carried the bulk of your excess weight all influence the potential for your skin to recoil to normal tone once you near your ideal weight. In the average patient, there is often an excess of body skin and fatty tissue. In the area of the belly and back, this excess of abdominal apron skin may be appropriately treated using procedures such as an *abdominoplasty* or *panniculectomy*. In more extreme excess skin situations, especially where the excess is circular in nature, involving the belly, hips, back, buttocks, and outer thighs, a more extensive procedure is available. This procedure is called a *belt lipectomy* and is like a face-lift for the torso. Both males and females may have excessive hanging breast tissue that can be reconstructed during a *breast lift* procedure. Some patients will have hanging tissue of the upper arms called "bat wings," which can be removed during a procedure called *brachioplasty*. Some patients will choose to undergo a *thigh lift* for the removal of the hanging folds of skin on their inner and outer thighs. Brachioplasty and thigh lift procedures are not usually "favorite" procedures of plastic surgeons, as there are no natural folds in these areas in which to hide the long scars.

In any case, make sure that you choose your plastic or reconstructive surgeon as wisely as you chose your bariatric surgeon. Make sure that your plastic surgeon is recognized by the American Board of Plastic Surgery as board certified. It is also important to know that your plastic surgeon has *regularly* performed the procedure you are considering, and it is one of his or her specialties. It is key that the plastic surgeon is familiar with the specific challenges that weight-loss surgery patients present, as our considerable amount of excess skin can be more difficult to reconstruct.

As I approached my goal weight, even regular exercise had not reduced the apron of skin hanging from my abdomen. Although this excess skin didn't medically compromise my life, I was unhappy with the way it looked. My surgeon performed an extended abdominoplasty panniculectomy, in which the lower abdominal incision runs about six inches past each of my hip bones. This allowed my surgeon to excise excess skin from my flanks in addition to my front belly area. This is the most common reconstructive procedure performed after weight-loss surgery. My abdominal reconstruction was considered cosmetic and was not a covered benefit of my insurance.

If you are considering reconstructive surgery once you have lost your weight, make sure that you visit your dermatologist if you suffer from any infections or rashes in your folds of skin, so that these problems can be noted on your medical chart. This may help you to prove to your insurance company that skin removal is medically necessary in your case.

It is worth noting that a new specialty in the field of plastic surgery is developing as our population of post-operative patients grows and requires skin removal unlike that of the *normal* population seeking plastic surgery.

J. Peter Rubin, M.D., is the founder and director of the Life After Weight Loss Program at the University of Pittsburgh Medical Center. He is nationally recognized in the rapidly evolving area of *post–bariatric surgery plastic and reconstructive surgery*. Dr. Rubin's technical skill, surgical innovation, and techniques in dealing with the typically large panels of hanging skin after massive weight loss have made him a leader in bringing these new developments into practice.

Dr. Alan Pillersdorf is another plastic/reconstructive surgeon who in addition to his regular practice has a passion for helping those who have fought to conquer morbid obesity. He has told me that he feels it is important to help bariatric post-ops to have a new body from which to enjoy their new life. In addition to his wonderful heart, he possesses a fine hand for detail in many of the more difficult procedures we seek. His practice is located in Royal Palm Beach, Florida.

It is my opinion that skin reduction operations of the upper arms and thighs should only be considered in the most extreme cases, and your surgeon should be chosen very carefully. These procedures are not commonplace in the average plastic surgeon's office, and given the difficulty in achieving even minimally aesthetically pleasing results with those who are the *most* practiced in this procedure, make sure that any surgeon you consider has at least a few of these under his belt. Make certain you have viewed these long thick rather awkward scars in person and that they are worth the tradeoff for you.

Ask to see photos of actual patient results of the surgeries you need or desire. I find that many people who have had a bariatric procedure followed by skin removal are willing to show you their scars. I would not consider a surgeon for any procedure before seeing his work on a patient with skin patterns similar to what I was bringing to the table.

I am 10 days post-op and cry when I see Burger King commercials on TV. What have I done to myself?

You haven't healed enough to be able to eat anything even resembling food, you are totally exhausted from your surgery, and your emotions are out of control—so it is not out of the question that you would sit around thinking how much you miss your old best friend, food. At this point you haven't lost a measurable amount of weight *and* you can't eat, so you have nothing. Once you have lost 65 or so pounds, you won't care as much about food, and by then you will be able to eat a little and won't think about what you are missing. Hang in there; I promise that it gets much, much better. I understand that it is terrible right now, but that will soon change and you will be able to laugh about the thought of crying over pictures of a Whopper! Soon you will reach that defining moment where the scale tips just enough in your favor for you to understand the meaning of "Nothing tastes as good as thin feels," and then it really gets exciting.

I am only a week post-op and I can drink an entire protein shake. Have I stretched out my pouch?

You cannot stretch out your pouch with liquids. It is simply impossible. It pours in and dribbles out. If you are sipping slowly, it is smoothly running in and out of your pouch. Even if the drain in the sink is half closed, the liquid won't back up as long as you are pouring it in gradually. Once you start eating more solid foods, like shrimp or chicken, you will see just how small your pouch is and that it is intact.

I am two months post-op and I have only lost 38 pounds. I am nervous and upset most of the time, as I am afraid that I will be the only one who this surgery doesn't work for. Does anyone else have these feelings?

Calm down and take a deep breath. You are just getting to the point where you have recovered from major surgery. Losing 38 pounds in two months is fantastic. We all have those moments when we think that we are the only one who isn't going to lose weight—that is normal considering our pitiful track records of losing weight and keeping it off. Some of us are faster losers from the start; others are slow and steady. Most of us even out over the course of that first year to similar totals. Don't put any added stress on yourself. Just remember to keep away from the carbs, start being aware of getting in more protein each day, start moving toward drinking 64 ounces of water a day, move around a little, and you will get there.

I am five months post-op and when I was washing my hair this morning, my fingers were completely tangled with hair that had fallen out. Help! What should I do?

I also lost what seemed to be a lot of hair during my fifth post-op month. It started out slowly and increased until I was in panic mode, running out and buying Biotin and adding a second 50-gram protein shake to my diet. I have a very knowledgeable dermatologist and he assured me that almost everyone who has a major operation would notice increased hair shedding for a few months afterward. On top of the shock of the surgery, our food intake plummets and we essentially develop protein malnutrition. The body then attempts to reserve protein by shifting the growing hairs into a resting phase. Massive hair shedding can occur two to three months later and even the remaining hair can be pulled out by the roots fairly easily. Once we rebound and begin to eat more protein, the condition reverses itself. For those of you who are considering this surgery, it is alarming seeing the hair in your drain. But it does grow back. By the end of my seventh post-op month, I had a head full of one-inch sprouts peeking through my longer hair! I am not trying to discount the impact of this hair loss, but it is temporary and does start to grow back very quickly. Fortunately it occurred at the time when I had lost enough weight and didn't focus as much on the hair loss. Friends weren't looking at my hair—they were noticing my incredible shrinking body. I took the opportunity to have a makeover and had my hairdresser give me a new, stylish, shorter look that I would never have tried at 278 pounds.

While initial hair shedding cannot be avoided, we can influence how fast it grows back with the help of dietary supplements.

I understand the impact of hair loss on our early journey and how upsetting it is. I cried many mornings over the hair in my shower drain and the sight of my scalp showing through my thinning hair on top of my head and in front.

I wanted to offer something more than a "don't worry about it—it's just hair" along with a bottle of Biotin. I made it a priority to work with a nutraceutical and nutrient scientist to create Journey Essentials Hair Balance Capsules, which is a nutrient boost for hair, nails, and skin. Hair Balance is a proprietary formulation of vitamins and botanically derived components that combines the power of methylsulfonylmethane (MSM)—a natural ingredient that allows hair to grow longer and faster by increasing the length of the hair cycle—with zinc, Biotin, and pantothenic acid into a potent hair-loss treatment regimen. Our feedback has been all positive, with many of you sending us photos of your long nails and improved hair status.

I've used it for months and am blown away by the increase in my hair and nail growth. While it will not grow hair where there was none, it will speed up the hair cycle and increase growth of what we have. The only negative is that I have to have my gray roots colored more often—but I'll happily take the trade-off.

I'm almost one year out . . . when does your self-image change? I am happy to be 165 pounds instead of 310, but I still see nothing but fat when I look in the mirror.

This is a common feeling that echoes in our monthly support group meetings. I'm sure it has a lot to do with a lifetime of seeing ourselves in a negative light, and as quickly as we all lose weight, our minds just don't have enough time to adjust to the physical change. We still see ourselves as fat because we are still the same person on the inside, looking at the world through the same eyes and anticipating certain behaviors from others. Now that we are wearing size 10 clothes, we realize that we aren't supermodels, we are real women and men, with curves, lumps, and wrinkles, and we are disappointed instead of being proud of our amazing success. I compare myself to photos of my girlfriends rather than the girls in the magazines to better center myself. This weight comes off so fast that we expect miracles, and if our life isn't suddenly transformed, we start to feel as if we are failures. Keep focusing on the great things that are happening for you, affirm your successes, celebrate every new step you have the courage to take, and you will find that it is so easy to love yourself.

Do I have to take multivitamins, iron, B_{12}, and calcium forever?

In one word, yes.

We have surgically changed the anatomy of how we eat and process our food and must be personally responsible for making up for essential nutrients we can no longer eat or absorb. When we don't pay attention, bad things can happen.

Just a short note to say hello as I am lying in the hospital starting iron infusions. Please remember to take your vitamins. Whether you are one, two, five, or eight years post-op . . . suck it up and take 'em, or you'll be in the same boat!

—Glen Blind, nine-year RNY (2003)
maintaining a 300-plus-pound weight loss

According to bariatric experts, the condition of morbid obesity is usually already accompanied by dietary vitamin and mineral deficiencies; many of us had deficiencies that went undetected before having surgery. Following surgery, gastric bypass patients typically experience additional deficiencies, because the procedure induces a state of semi-starvation; we simply cannot ingest enough food to provide sufficient nutrition. The new twist is that experts feel that post-operative deficiencies occur largely because patients do not have nutrient-rich diets and do not take vitamin and mineral supplements. We often cause our own deficiencies because we don't do as we are told.

The typical gastric bypass procedure reduces fat absorption and, along with it, the absorption of fat-soluble vitamins, such as beta-carotene, vitamin D, vitamin E, and vitamin K. Protein deficiencies, the inability to eat red meat, and the reduced use of dairy products, combined with a drastic reduction in the amounts of fruits and vegetables eaten, may be responsible for low blood and tissue levels of calcium, iron, magnesium, potassium, and zinc. The limited use of dairy products and/or lactose intolerance further reduces the calcium position of the bariatric patient. The lack of digestive enzymes and stomach acids coming into contact with food also plays an important role in mineral absorption.

Once we've had bariatric surgery, it's important for us to follow up with our surgical team and then after with our primary physician to remain vital. Our lab values must be monitored, and any problems remedied before they affect quality of life. Lifelong usage of multivitamin, iron, B vitamins, and calcium supplements are not simply suggestions but are mandatory following bariatric surgery.

When I had surgery in 2001, it was commonplace for surgeons to tell their patients to take a couple of daily Flintstones paired with three or four Tums. I quickly noticed that the patients a few months ahead of me were practically bald and looked tired, with dark under-eye circles. When I reached the six-month stage, I remember the day that my friend Ronni told me that even though I was in her home for only a few minutes, she was able to sweep up a disturbingly large pile of my long dark hair from her white tile floors. Within weeks I could see through to my scalp on the top and front of my head—and it was devastating. I never tied my hair loss to my lack of good nutrients, and for more than eighteen months the baldness did not improve.

It wasn't until eating became less of an effort that the importance of taking my supplements registered with me. I started using a single product—bariatric vitamin supplement in a capsule form—and things began turning around for me within weeks. Once I was able to keep a decent schedule for taking my supplements, my hair returned and energy levels improved. I chose to have this surgery to be healthy and fit, yet for almost two years I lackadaisically took vitamins designed for a 40-pound child.

Over the years I've seen more and more of my surgical contemporaries with severe symptoms pointing to nutrient deficiencies, most notably anemia, but in some cases even seizures and neurological damage from lack of nutrient compliance and absorption. I don't know if surgical programs fail to stress the consequences of poor vitamin habits or if patients just don't think it will happen to them, but studies show that as many as 78 percent of patients do not take any supplements at all. It is crucial to come up with a combination that works for your lifestyle that you will be able to adhere to. If you do not take good-quality supplements, you *will* eventually suffer from deficiencies. Some deficiencies cause irreversible damage—this is nothing to take lightly.

I didn't know I had severe vitamin D and calcium deficiencies until I snapped my leg in a motorcycle accident in Key West in 2008. The orthopedic surgeon told me that when he placed the plate and screws to fix my fracture, my bones were like a stick of butter. For years after my surgery, my vitamin D deficiency had gone unnoticed; I was not taking my supplements as required, and it is also likely I had the deficiency prior to my surgery, as the *25-hydroxy vitamin D test* is not automatically run with standard blood lab tests. This was my awakening. I now know not only how important it is to take supplements but also to choose those that are specifically designed for our altered digestive systems. It's not which vitamins we take, it's how much our bodies absorb and how we make it a task we can complete daily. I wish I had this epiphany when I was newly post-op.

I've worked with specialists to develop the Journey Bariatric and Journey Essentials lines of dietary supplements. We based the principles of these top-quality supplements on all that I have gone through. I acknowledge not taking all my supplements; no matter how good my intentions, I was unable to manage all those different bottles of bariatric vitamins on schedule. I felt guilty about my hair loss, I dragged for years from low iron, and I had soft bones and fractured a leg because of my calcium deficiency, and all because I loathed the giant chalky chewable tablets and didn't take all of them every day. I know there are millions of you who are just like me—you want to take supplements but are ashamed you're not taking them, assuming you're the only one failing. What was available on the market unintentionally set us up for compliance failure.

So we came up with Journey Bariatric Multiformula—an all-in-one formulation that is simple to use: three capsules or melts, twice daily. For those who already have deficiencies, there are separate iron, vitamin D_3, and calcium in forms that make scientific sense for our body modifications. For those who do not want capsules, Journey uses soft melt technology for smooth-textured, small, unobtrusive tablets with true natural flavorings and colorings. We chose a gentle form of iron called Ferrochel® that is highly efficient yet does not cause the burning and constipation of other forms of iron. This is the iron recommended by many hematologists for those with deficiencies severe enough to warrant IV iron infusions that many of my friends, including Glen, have endured.

We have also created Journey Hair Balance, which supports faster growth of our hair and nails—amazing what a little of the latest science can do. Since I know how devastating hair loss can be, we created a formulation that backs growth at the first opportunity.

Don't make the mistakes I made early on—as soon as you are feeling somewhat better after returning home from your surgery and are eating soft foods, start taking good-quality supplements. The average patient has a lot of difficulty in adhering to the standby chewable vitamin program that requires multiple products to be taken at different times throughout the day. I too have always struggled with compliance, but the best intentions in the world cannot overcome our potential for deficiency.

The best supplements for you are ones that you can commit to take every day. I created Journey because we're truly on this journey together.

What kind of calcium is the best one for us to take, calcium carbonate or calcium citrate?

While calcium carbonate is adequate for the average person to use to supplement their diet, calcium citrate is a better form of calcium for gastric bypass patients, as we no longer have the necessary stomach acids in our pouches or bypassed intestines to facilitate calcium carbonate absorption.

The National Institutes of Health, in its Consensus Statement regarding Optimal Calcium Uptake, clearly makes the case for calcium citrate.

Absorption of one form of calcium supplementation, calcium carbonate, is impaired in fasted individuals who have an absence of gastric acid. Alternatively, calcium supplementation in the form of calcium citrate does not require gastric acid for optimal absorption and thus could be considered in individuals with reduced gastric acid production.

Additionally, the University of Pittsburgh Medical Center published the results of a study called: "Bone Loss Associated with Weight Loss After Stomach Reduction Surgery." Dr. Penelope Coates, M.D., postdoctoral fellow at the University of Pittsburgh Medical Center's Osteoporosis Prevention and Treatment Center, has discovered that women and men who have stomach reduction surgery to lose weight may be losing bone mass even when they take daily calcium supplements, putting them at risk for osteoporosis and bone fracture.

We have been recommending that people take 1000 mg calcium citrate daily because we were concerned that calcium carbonate would not be absorbed after the surgery. The calcium in Tums is calcium carbonate. Our patients were taking a variety of supplements but have largely switched to calcium citrate.

How can I swallow my pills when I can't drink enough water to get them down?

Immediately post-op I would bury my pills in a spoonful of sugar-free Jell-O instant pudding. I kept a bowl in the refrigerator just for taking pills. Something about the smooth, thick texture made it easier for me than water, since I could only take baby sips of water. The small pills I could take whole; larger ones I would cut into quarters.

What's so important about exercise?

When you have a gastric bypass, you lose weight because the amount of food energy that you eat is much less than what your body needs to operate. It has to make up the difference by burning reserves. If you do not exercise daily, your body will metabolize your unused muscle, and you will lose muscle mass and strength. Daily aerobic exercise for at least 20 minutes will communicate to your body that you want to use your muscles, and force it to burn the fat instead. The idea of having this operation is to become slender and healthy, not scrawny and weak. If you lose most of your excess fat, and retain most of your muscles, imagine how much power and energy you will have to enjoy your reclaimed life. Walk, skip, jump, dance around the house—move!

When can I have a few vegetables? I am craving some salad.

Once you have gotten through the initial few weeks of intense healing and have started to get comfortable with eating again, it is all right to add in a few bites of very-low-carbohydrate vegetables after you eat your needed protein. Once I was two months post-op and was doing well in eating my small portions of shrimp salad and softly cooked salmon, I added a small handful of lightly dressed baby salad greens to my plate and would chew a tender leaf with a few of my bites of food. I would cook a few baby spinach leaves with my shrimp in a little garlic and olive oil; the spinach shreds would add moisture to the mouthful and make it even easier to eat. Just make sure that you choose low-carb vegetables, and that you eat four or five bites of protein for every one bite of vegetable. A tablespoon of sautéed, seasoned spinach or a few bites of baby lettuce leaves add less than one gram of carbohydrate to your daily tally, so even surgeons with the strictest nutritional regimen would agree with this one.

Is it all right to drink soda?

No, don't drink soda; even diet soda is a blast back to your old life. Once your stomach and intestines are healed from your surgery, drinking a diet soda won't explode your pouch or anything as dramatic. However, it isn't always just physical damage we are trying to avoid. People who struggle and gain back weight or never reach their goals usually have this in common: drinking with meals, in particular soda. We are trying to develop new healthy habits, and soda is a link back to bad habits and the foods like Doritos, chips, and fries. Leave all of it in your past.

Ever since my surgery I have a gurgling sound when I swallow and terrible burping when I eat or drink. Is something wrong?

The gurgles or burps in your esophagus and stomach are normal. You used to have a big stomach bag for all that air and food to roll around in. Now that your stomach is a tiny pouch, there just isn't much space for the air you were unaware that you were gulping. Just be more conscious of taking in extra air while you are eating and drinking and it will lessen.

Once in a while a food will make me sick but when I throw it up, there is so much spit and mucus. Does this happen to everyone?

When we eat something that our stomach cannot handle, the problem gets compounded when the undigested food is quickly dumped into our intestines. The intestines draw water from the bloodstream in an attempt to dilute the offending food. This creates the excessive mucus and slime. I find that this happens if I eat too fast, don't chew well, or continue to eat when I am already full, so it definitely serves as negative reinforcement for me!

What was the thing that surprised you the most in the first year of your weight loss?

My husband's daughter, Dione, had mailed me a pair of size-eight Calvin Klein capri jeans and a disposable camera in a package that were waiting for me when I came home from the hospital. I started to cry when I saw the tiny little pants and held them up to my huge body. I looked at my husband and just shook my head and laughed to hide the pain in knowing that I would never fit into those pants. There was a letter in the package, instructing me to have Ty take a photo of me right then and again on each month's anniversary date for the next year, so that I would never forget what I went through. There was no way that I wanted to have my picture taken in my huge flowered robe with my bloated belly, but my husband kept on it and I finally gave in. Every month on the 11th, there he was with that camera to take my picture. After he took the last picture, I dropped off the camera, but I didn't pick up the photos for several months.

I actually have two things that surprised me during the first year of my weight loss. The first is that I actually lost enough weight to slip into those size-eight pants. I am always particularly humble while wearing them.

The second is that it is incredible to have a photo journal of my progress during those months of losing such a large amount of weight. It was so thoughtful, and it was not something that I would have ever done on my own. It took me a while to get up the courage to pick up the pictures—the reality of what I looked like was truly shocking—but I am so proud of all that I went through to get where I am right now.

Note: While this is a great suggestion, don't pose for your photos in your underwear, as I did, or even worse, without any clothes, as you won't be able to show the photos to anyone or put them in your book!

The way I understand it, there are people who have a higher risk going into surgery and those with a lower risk. Is there anything that I can do to lower my surgical risk?

Remember that in order to even be considered for a bariatric procedure, the risk to your life of having the surgery must be smaller than your risk of not having surgery. However, it is very smart of you to think in terms of minimizing those risks that are within your control.

Your choice of surgeon gives you the greatest ability to manage your surgical risk. Some surgeons have better statistical outcomes than others in addition to having performed more procedures. In my opinion, it is essential to choose a surgical team that the American Society for Bariatric Surgery (ASBS) has identified as an ASBS Bariatric Surgery Center of Excellence. These are the top surgeons as identified by their own member organization. Personally I would not want to be a doctor's tenth patient, nor would I want my bariatric surgery to be his only one for the month.

It is preferable to have your bariatric surgery performed as a minimally invasive, laparoscopic procedure, than as an open-incision surgery, as the minimally invasive approach is just as effective with fewer complications. The only people who might not agree with this assessment would be surgeons who are not trained to perform the procedures via this highly specialized mode of access to the organs. If a surgeon is qualified to do the procedure both ways, his first choice, as long as you meet the physical criteria, will be the laparoscopic method. There are many very good surgeons who obtain excellent results via an open incision, but the laparoscopic method will decrease the likelihood of wound infections; lower post-operative pain; and, in many cases, shorten the hospital stay.

Get in the best physical shape possible right before your surgery. Making the healthy lifestyle changes of increasing activity, taking vitamins, and eating a healthy diet before surgery will put you in the best possible condition for major surgery and general anesthesia. Do not gain weight before your operation. You don't need large *last meals,* as there truly is nothing that you cannot have a small taste of at a later time. A weight gain just prior to surgery increases your risk factor and is contrary to the good choices we have made to diminish controllable risk.

Is there a higher rate of divorce once a spouse has had weight-loss surgery?

If you are in a good relationship before you have a bariatric procedure, you should find yourself in a good relationship after the weight loss. There is definite potential for difficulties any time one person goes through such unprecedented change and the other does not, but if you are in a mutually responsible relationship, you should be able to endure the change and continue to grow.

Now, bad relationships are another story. I know many people who are in nearly intolerable situations but, due to their obesity, feel as if there is no choice. They feel hopeless, unloved, and undeserving, and lack self-esteem—in some cases their partner both suggests and reinforces these negatives. I think that some people who enter into relationships with the obese are drawn to and actively seek those who won't make the typical demands of a mutual relationship and generally suppress their own needs or view them as insignificant. Once the obese partner loses weight, feels good about himself or herself and feels deserving of happiness, he or she no longer wants to stay in the unfulfilling situation. However they sometimes remain victims of their own weight even once it's gone.

Weight-loss surgery doesn't cause divorces; bad relationships cause breakups and divorce. If one person suddenly feels good about himself or herself and the other person cannot find joy in this new-found light, the relationship was not a nurturing partnership.

I hate to say it, but my girlfriends seem jealous that I am not the biggest one in our group anymore. No one really talks about it, but how common is it to lose your friends? I can speak to this subject personally as I lost what I considered to be two very strong friendships after my weight loss. People become friends because of commonality, and when someone loses a large amount of weight, his or her entire life changes, the dynamic of relationships change, and friendships don't always survive.

My best friend of more than 17 years is no longer a part of my life. I now sadly recognize that she has had a life filled with drama, and I provided her with instant self-esteem. No matter how unpleasant her saga became, she could always take solace in the fact that she was thin and attractive. When I lost weight, my life changed and was suddenly filled with everything good. While on the surface she seemed truly happy for me, my new life emphasized the lack of good in hers. I look back on our years together and recognize that she was frequently malevolent toward others in her life who were happy. The loss of this friendship hurts me deeply as I thought we would literally be friends for life through thick and thin.

I lost the friendship of a good weight-loss-surgery friend as well. We had our surgery at the same time and were both thrilled to slide down the scale to our goal weights. She was not a model for good post-operative nutrition and I was the one *who wrote the book,* but sneaking chocolate and eating bread doesn't affect *early* weight loss and I overlooked our differences. When we turned the corner at the four-year mark she was back to eating the same foods that had made her morbidly obese, but in smaller quantities. No matter how much I tried to help her, she seemed both undedicated and unable to make the changes needed to take back control of her weight. She needed professional help for her emotional eating issues. Growing out of size-fourteen clothes when she had once been so proud to wear a size eight only drove her deeper into denial, and her pre-operative misery and cynicism returned. I had once been a positive influence, but good intentions turned into nagging and strained our relationship even more. I can't let go of the fact that she has squandered her opportunity yet still laughs at those who believe in support groups and accountability, so it's better that we no longer be friends.

Morbidly obese people often take what we can get in terms of relationships, because we are not happy with who we are. This changes as we lose weight, and the casualties are sometimes those we thought were good friends. Relationships come and go in life, and it is a natural progression to have friends who fit not only who we are but who we have become.

I have extreme fatigue and exhaustion. I switched to more appropriate bariatric vitamins and added B_{12} to my schedule even though my lab results looked fine to my primary care physician. I get enough protein and drink my fluids. It has been three years since my RNY surgery and it often takes everything I've got to get up and do what needs to be done. I have a post-op friend about a year ahead of me and she often complains of being tired too. Is this just a reality I need to accept?

Make sure that you are getting complete lab work done that includes tests for *ferritin,* which assays *stored iron* in the body (blood iron levels may remain at normal levels while we deplete stored iron—anemia is easier to catch early than treat later), and *all B vitamins* (not just B_{12}), and a *thyroid panel including TSH* levels (thyroid-stimulating hormone regulates metabolism). These are not necessarily standard tests but can sometimes provide clues to the source of symptoms for treatment. We had bariatric surgery to be healthy, and fatigue is not a necessary consequence of this surgery.

There is a point at which we no longer return to our bariatric surgeon for aftercare, so it is important that we have a primary care doctor willing to deal with our health in terms of our weight-loss surgery. We have absorption issues and special nutritional needs that must be monitored, and while it's important that we know how to manage our own health needs, we need a good PCP as well. If your primary care physician is unaware of details of your surgery or is unwilling to learn, find another who is.

At the four-year post-op mark, I started having a hard time keeping my head up while working at my computer late at night, but I was sleeping later as well. My weight increased without a change in my diet, and I noticed excessive hair on the bathroom floor. I chose to blame myself and cut way back on my calories, but I continued to slowly gain. After several months of this, I went to my primary care doctor in tears. He asked me a few questions and felt certain that the culprit was once again my thyroid, or what remained of it. A lab test for thyroid-stimulating hormone showed a level off the charts when it should have been near zero. My metabolism had practically stopped, and no amount of cutting back on calories was going to jump-start my energy levels. In addition, my ferritin iron level showed a decrease, pointing toward anemia.

My thyroid levels have been stabilized with daily Synthroid, and without a change in diet I dropped the weight I'd gained in six weeks and my hair stopped falling out.

I now take Journey Bariatric Multiformula Capsules—three small capsules in the morning and three in the afternoon or evening have kept my lab values strong—plus a Journey Essential Gentle Iron in a natural grape-flavored melt tablet. Journey uses a patented, highly specialized iron called Ferrochel that does not prevent calcium intake, so it's okay that it's contained in the same formula. The iron in Journey is the form often recommended by hematologists when they are treating post-op iron deficiencies, and it's both extremely efficient and safe. Low iron can leave us feeling drained and fatigued—make sure you keep up with your lab values to prevent this common deficiency, along with any others that can pop up.

I am too scared to have the gastric bypass RNY procedure so I am having a Lap-Band procedure. How can I make sure I am successful even though the weight loss isn't as dramatic?

In order to get to a healthy weight using the Lap-Band as your tool of choice, it is important for you to eat as if you had had the more involved RNY surgery. Lap-Band surgery is less physically restrictive, which is why some choose it, thinking it will somehow be easier; this is far from true. Even though the procedure is less involved in that there is no cutting or rerouting of organs, you are still altering your body by means of a serious surgical procedure, and Lap-Band surgery actually demands greater participation in making dietary changes.

My surgeon has not given me a clear outline as to what I can eat when I return home from my surgery. I have one page telling me to slowly add solid foods to my diet. Shouldn't I have more information?

When you get home from the hospital, you will start a nutrition plan to slowly advance you from a liquid diet to a solid diet. This progression is similar for all bariatric procedures except for patients who have special dietary needs due to outside medical situations or complications. There can be large differences in the length of time you spend in each stage as allowed by different RNY and Lap-Band surgeons; some surgeons are still extremely conservative while others have more up-to-date plans for moving forward into soft foods. While I am not a doctor, I have personally experienced bariatric surgery and understand that the point of a slow transition is to avoid vomiting and not stress the newly created pouch or potentially block the openings.

I have made lists of allowable foods for these stages and meals that you can reference for ideas on pages 103–111. A good way to understand my position is to recognize that just because someone *says* that you can eat chicken, it doesn't mean you actually can. I know that these first few transition weeks after surgery are very difficult as we don't feel well, we are scared, we don't know what to eat, and on top of everything, nothing tastes right. This is why the new chapter on food progressions will be helpful to you.

I am tired of being disappointed every time I get on the scale, but the weight is coming off so slowly. How can I stay positive when I still have so much weight to lose?
The weight is coming off slowly compared to what? Whose time frame are you setting your goal by? This is not an end-oriented race; it is an ongoing process. You will lose at your own pace, and the final goal is not to arrive at a particular weight by an arbitrary time, but to develop a new way of eating that you can live with for the rest of your life.

A good way to remain positive is to set attainable and realistic goals for your journey. We need to set small short-term goals, and treat ourselves with kindness when we get there. Many of us establish a goal of losing 50 pounds in three months, 75 pounds in six months, or 100 pounds in 12 months, and this is the epitome of a negative goal. I did this also as it is human nature for us to be impatient. Qualifying the weight loss with a time frame sets us up for a potential or even probable failure. When we lose 50 pounds in four months rather than three we turn what should be a happy affirmation into a negative.

Set a goal of rewarding yourself with a pair of earrings or a new workout outfit when you lose your first 50 pounds. This goal is 100 percent positive and there is no way to ruin your happiness in attaining it. You reach your goal; you lose 50 pounds, you are happy, and you celebrate your success with something to show off your slimmer self. We can't lose when we set positive goals and reward ourselves when we simply accomplish them.

Will our higher-protein lifestyle put us at risk for kidney problems?

Research has shown that a higher-protein diet has no effect on kidney function for people with normal kidneys. Protein does not cause renal disorders. Note that it is proven that type 2 diabetes, which is associated with obesity, has become one of the most common identifyable causes of kidney disease. Extra body mass and circulating blood puts a huge load on your kidneys, sometimes leading to kidney disorders. Losing weight helps your kidneys by removing the extra work they have to do.

When we get our lab results, many of us hear that our protein levels are *good* and think that this means that we are eating enough protein, when this actually means that our kidneys are functioning properly.

I used to drink socially before I had my surgery. Is it safe for me to drink a beer when I am out with my friends? Do you drink?

Many of us have questions about whether or not to drink alcoholic beverages after our bariatric surgery. You shouldn't even consider having a drink of alcohol unless you have discussed it with your surgeon and have his or her approval. I don't believe that any surgeon would allow an alcoholic beverage for anyone who is less than a full year out of surgery.

With the new configuration of our organs, alcohol is not digested before being dumped into our intestines; this increases the level of alcohol directly entering our bloodstream. We always have to be careful when drinking any alcohol as its effects can be greatly amplified. After bariatric surgery we are cheap dates. Don't drink when you are out alone or where your safety could be compromised should you be overcome by the effects of alcohol; never drive if you've had any alcohol.

In addition to the increased absorption of the alcohol, we also must carefully watch sugar levels and avoid carbonation. Most cocktails and mixed drinks use sugary mixers or sweetened fruit bases, and will quickly make us sick. We need to step back and really think when faced with an alcohol-related choice. I have attended social events for and with bariatric patients and watched in horror while surgical post-ops ordered frozen strawberry margaritas and mudslides with whipped cream!

I will from time to time drink an alcoholic beverage when we are out, but I am very careful about the ingredients. When I was one year post-op, I would order a wine cocktail consisting of a tall glass of ice filled to half with white wine, the rest with club soda, with a squeeze of fresh lemon and orange (the ice quickly flattens the carbonation of the club soda). Flavored vodkas do not contain any sugar but are infused with fruit essence; I love Stoli Razberi with lots of club soda and fresh lime. When we are out with our motorcycle friends I will *hang on to* a bottle of Michelob Ultra or Miller Lite and take an occasional sip; it's low in carbs and calories. I am always aware of what I am drinking and am very careful; I want to have fun but I want to be safe and not compromise my health.

I am tired of well-meaning friends and family telling me that I could lose if I would only eat less and exercise more. My mother keeps bringing up the Jenny Craig ads with Kirstie Alley. I have dieted myself up to over 300 pounds. Why does my family think I am weak and simply lack self-control?
Many of us have been told that we are failures for considering weight-loss surgery. We are told that we could realize long-term weight loss if only we had more willpower or exercised more. The problem is that most normal-size people can't relate to our obesity problem.

It is documented that commercial diet programs, behavioral modification programs, and exercise programs fail at least 95 percent of the time. Society assumes that severely obese people have only themselves to blame. However, most of us are successful in most aspects of our careers and personal lives. We are not lazy people without discipline; we are successful people who are able to accomplish many goals in life, but have been unable to find a solution to our weight problem. Just as it is impossible to change our height or eye color, it is not possible for many of us to overcome the genetics or the emotional eating disorders that lead to becoming more than 100 pounds overweight without the added tool of bariatric surgery backed by appropriate counseling.

We are not failures for seeking surgical help, as it takes courage and commitment to health to even consider bariatric surgery. We all know that this isn't the easy way out. It takes great courage to embark on a journey of this magnitude.

I'm always too busy to eat breakfast, and I'm not a morning person. Will this hurt my overall weight loss?

Severe calorie restriction creates a situation that tells your body it's starving! Your body responds by slowing your metabolism in order to hold on to existing stored energy. In addition, if the food shortage continues, you'll begin to burn fat *and* muscle tissue, which will further lower your metabolic rate. Don't skip meals.

We don't plan to fail, we just fail to plan! I'm not a morning person, but rather than change, I work around it. Keep a bag of Inspire Caramel Latte whey protein isolate drink mix in your desk drawer to add to your nine A.M. coffee. Have several Believe Mocha Latte or Smooth Chai Tea bottled protein drinks in your refrigerator so you can grab one to drink in your car on the way out the door in the morning. Starting your day off with protein will help keep your metabolism working at full power and in your favor. A great benefit for a little effort!

You talk about this surgery and never mention anything bad happening to anyone. Are there any people you know who have had problems after their initial bariatric surgery?

I know a lot of people who are not successful with their surgery, but it is a reasonably small percentage of all procedures, and many problems are minor and quickly remedied.

A large percentage of negative issues are caused by noncompliance or simply not listening, and before people know it they have a situation they can't dig their way out of. The problems include anemia, hair loss, slow weight loss and long stalls, and weight gain—things that could have been avoided with good nutrition, plenty of protein, taking vitamins every day, following up with doctor's after-care, and attending support groups. These are generally the patients who fail to understand that they have a responsibility to follow a program once they have had surgery to treat their obesity, and that lasting weight loss and good health are not automatic.

During the healing process a small percentage will develop a stricture, which is the narrowing of the surgically created opening. Once this is discovered, there is a fairly simple procedure to remedy the problem; the patient is put under light sedation and a scope is inserted down the throat with a balloon tip that expands to gently push back and stretch the tissue. I have not had this done, but those who have tell me that it is not as bad as it sounds and that the relief is immediate. Some need the procedure repeated several times, and of course this makes things difficult during the initial recovery phase, but there are usually no lasting effects.

I think that the most serious problem is in the handful of people I know who can't stop losing weight once they blow right through their goal on the way down. People often joke that they would like to have this problem, but I can assure them that it is not fun. Sometimes there is an underlying emotional problem that is contributing to the situation. One of my friends is under tremendous stress because her husband is an Army officer serving in Iraq. She has no desire to eat, and her only nutrients come from the few protein drinks she manages to force herself to drink each day. She has obtained psychological help as she knows that she must overcome her lack of desire for food in order to remain alive and healthy.

I have another friend who developed ulcers that caused her tre-mendous pain when she ate or even took a sip of water. Her weight became so dangerously low that she needed to have a peripherally inserted central catheter, or PICC line, which enables her to receive a constant supply of nourishment that is directly released into her blood, in order for her ulcers to be able to heal. She recently underwent a revision procedure to remove a portion of her ulcerated pouch. She is slowly approaching the corner as she has managed to gain several pounds since her second surgery by drinking one of our supplements with a very high concentration of protein. She is an amazing person, and throughout this ordeal she has remained positive and mentally strong. Her pouch has healed enough that she can once again eat a soft post-op diet and is doing very well.

Another friend who has gone from being morbidly obese to severely underweight has developed an attitude to food that is not unlike that of an anorexic. Even though she knows that she needs to consume more calories, she is actually unable to force herself to eat foods that are high in calories, or foods that are not fat free or essentially carbohydrate free. I encourage her to prepare egg custards using half-and-half, to use a little extra olive oil in cooking to add concentrated calories, and to eat many small meals throughout the day, but she is paralyzed with fear that she will be morbidly obese again.

A small percentage of people develop gallbladder problems or blockages after a rapid initial weight loss. Fortunately all that I know have undergone laparoscopic removal of the offending organ and have made a speedy recovery.

A few other friends have had intestinal twists or blockages, some requiring surgery. I understand that there is higher risk of this once someone has had weight-loss surgery, but that adhesions can develop any time the abdomen is entered for any surgical procedure.

To put this into perspective, there is small percentage of problems attached to having a bariatric procedure once you have made it out of the operating room. However, I would imagine that the same population of morbidly obese people would likely have a greater number of complications and medical problems due to their obesity if they had never lost weight as a result of having this surgery.

**Now that you have the benefit of almost eleven years
of "hands-on" experience since your surgery, what is
the best advice that you can give to someone having
bariatric surgery next week?**
This surgery is truly a medical miracle that can change your life, but
it doesn't do all the work for you. I don't think that anyone realizes
how difficult this procedure really is or just how devoted they will
have to be in order to stay slim and healthy for the rest of their life,
not just in the short term.

Very few professionals talk about the *not so insignificant* percentage of people who gain back substantial weight. Many are still considered a success by medical standards as they maintain as much as half
of their initial loss, but I don't think that anyone has this serious an
operation for a net loss of 50 pounds. I know people who had their
surgery when I did that are over 200 pounds again. They are gaining
weight because they bend rules that they never respected in the first
place. In addition, many have eating disorders that were not treated
in tandem with their morbid obesity.

What many gainers have in common is that they never turned
over their life to this surgery. They looked at it as a one-year diet that
would give them a fresh start, and figured that they would be able
to control their habits once they lost the weight. Within eight to ten
months they are already eating trigger foods without paying attention
to protein and carbohydrates, and often washing it all down with
diet or even regular soda. They are always hungry because of the
"yummy" bread, crackers, chips, and pasta carbs they justify eating,
and know that they don't get sick on sugar because they pushed the
line early on and discovered that if they only ate a small amount at
a time, they only got "a little" sick. They are out of control because
they never had control but thought the surgery would provide it for
them with minimal participation.

My advice is to go into this surgery knowing that it is going to take a lot of work and dedication to your health. Know the rules, identify the boundaries, and be prepared to live without crossing them for the rest of your life. Find healthy and delicious foods that are allowed in your new life that you love as much as the bad foods from your old life.

Finally, understand that this surgery has great potential for creating happiness if you train yourself to look for the good things as they unfold instead of the bad. Don't be sad about the things you can't eat, be happy with the things you *can* eat while enjoying a slimmer and healthier body. Learn to love your new life, but even more important, learn to love yourself!

There is so much misinformation out there and everyone wants to tell me about the bad things that happened to their friend. Can you give me the basics of what I need to know?

I have a very accurate and informative message board where many of my most successful post-op friends gather almost daily and this is the list we put together as a group effort for the new folks having surgery. We call it Weight-Loss Surgery 101.

1. Never compare your journey or results to anyone else's.
2. Don't worry; you are not going to be the only person for whom this surgery does not work. Just do what you are supposed to and you will be a success.
3. Find palatable protein. There are many brands out there that will be so horrible that it will be difficult to drink them. However, there is no need to punish yourself, which is why the BariatricEating.com protein suggestions are so popular!
4. Don't kid yourself: this is major surgery and it will probably

hurt somewhat. This is why they provide us with pain management, just in case we need it.

5. Post-op depression is not uncommon. We are losing the comfort of our best friend—food—so depression is bound to raise its head if you've experienced it in the past.

6. You will recover much faster if you walk as much as you can.

7. Follow the post-op diet instructions. Do not accelerate your food progression.

8. In the weeks immediately after your procedure, your main job is healing.

9. When you start feeling better after your surgery, slowly add vitamins to your daily routine.

10. A year from now you won't remember the bad times as much as you will be happy with the results!

11. Once you have been released by your surgeon for solid foods as pureed or blended, keep it *very* moist.

12. If the food is consistently painful going down or you consistently throw it up, call your surgeon. If you are throwing up water or liquids, don't wait to call.

13. Address issues quickly and proactively. Get involved with your own aftercare.

14. Dehydration is serious! Drink at least 64 ounces of fluids a day, and more is better.

15. Find support with other weight-loss surgery post-ops who can relate. Message boards (especially BeforeAndAfterHelp .com), support meetings, whatever it is, just do it. Accountability is key.

16. Take *before* pictures. You will amaze yourself with what you see in pictures even if you *think* you don't see it looking in the mirror! There is no denying photographic proof!

17. When starting to eat again, remember you have the rest of your life to eat. In the big picture, two weeks on full liquids

isn't that long. Don't try to advance to more solid stages of food before your time.

18. Look at the big picture. It's not how much weight you've lost this week, it's how much weight you've lost overall.

19. Purchase early post-op supplies in small quantities; when you eat two ounces at a time, a small container of yogurt contains three portions.

20. Read this book over and over during your recovery, and join the companion positive support board. There are so many additional wonderful recipes, and it's full of people who talk the talk and walk the walk.

21. Make sure you use your early months to change your habits. Just because you can eat something without bad results, it doesn't mean you should.

22. You are not *lucky* if sugar doesn't make you sick. You are foolish for pushing the limits and will have eliminated a very important line of defense in the battle for control.

23. Know what you are eating. Read labels, and if any form of sugar is listed as one of the first five ingredients, it is not a good choice! High-fructose corn syrup, corn syrup, fructose, honey, maple syrup, and sucrose are all forms of sugar.

24. Nothing tastes as good as thin feels! Repeat that out loud when faced with a food challenge.

25. Do not drink with food. Once you take your first bite, unless you are choking, leave the beverage alone.

26. Immediately after your surgery things taste unbearably sweet for several weeks. Don't be alarmed by how your tastes have changed as your taste buds will eventually settle down.

27. There is more than one kind of weight-loss surgery. Make certain you know which surgery you are going to have, and never assume that everything you read or hear will be appropriate for your situation.

28. Once you and your surgeon have decided on your
    procedure, educate yourself on what is going to happen
    before, during, and after your surgery.
29. Resolve that you are going to follow your surgeon's
    instructions to the letter.
30. For maximum results, exercise is not an option, it's mandatory.

You and Ty have so much fun together, and I love hearing about your motorcycle rides and trips to Vegas. Do you know any single Harley-riding men who you could introduce me to? I am 35 and I suddenly find myself terrified of being alone, but even more terrified to open myself up for rejection as I have never really dated or been social.

We always have a good time, and we do have a couple of nice single male friends with Harleys! I know many women (and men) in your situation. Being overweight teaches some of us to hide. Many people who live with obesity have hidden for years. They have kept quiet in a crowd. They have spoken little at work. They sit and listen at family gatherings. If you are going to be out in the world, you are going to have to learn to be brave and have confidence in your new self. Just a small part of what you communicate is what you say; the rest comes through your actions.

I have a weight-loss surgery friend who is 35 and single; she has limited dating experience as she has been obese her entire adult life. Her problem now that she is slim is that she's not approachable. She is unhappy with her self-image and negative about her life, and she gripes about the bad things that "only happen to her." When we go out, she puts up a wall and lashes out at anyone who comes near, almost as if to hurt them before they can hurt her. She forgets that people don't penalize her for being the *fat girl* anymore. Until she begins to love herself, and look for the positives in life that exist all around her, happiness and someone to share it with will likely continue to elude her.

Smile, be friendly, make eye contact, and have confidence that people would actually want to know you and would enjoy what you would bring to a relationship. Rather than searching for someone, picture yourself as a magnet that will attract someone. There are nice people out there who will find you. Just remember that *the one* isn't going to knock on your door or suddenly appear on your couch, so you are going to have to be out there.

It has never been addressed in any group or support meetings I have attended, but people who have been obese all of their lives and suddenly find themselves inhabiting a thin body basically have to go through another sexual adolescence, and I imagine it is as difficult when you are 35 and single as when you were 17. Make sure you have either an online or live support group, as you are not the only one to face these issues and interacting with your group is a good first step in getting out more, meeting people, and overcoming these common concerns and fears.

My nutritionist doesn't want me using protein supplements; she would rather I get my protein from food. However, this doesn't seem to be the advice that everyone else is given. Why isn't it better to get my protein from food once I have had my surgery?
I bet that your nutritionist didn't have bariatric surgery, and I would venture to say that she is probably new, but that's okay as her advice obviously didn't sound right to you and threw out a red flag. It would be a great thing if after our surgery we were able to get all our nutrition from the foods that we eat. However, our bariatric surgery reduced our stomach size to effectively hold just a few ounces of food

at a time. So while in theory we should simply make healthy food choices for the rest of our life, the reality is that we can't fit enough healthy food in our small stomachs to get the nutrition we need.

One ounce of a protein food such as egg, chicken, or shrimp contains about 7 grams of protein. If our bodies needs 70 grams of protein a day, that means we would have to eat 10 ounces of egg, chicken, or shrimp. It would be physically difficult or impossible to do that, so we have to make up the difference with protein supplements. Early on we have to make up a larger difference between what we can eat and what we need, but even eleven years after my surgery, eating 10 ounces of protein daily is unreasonable, so I often start off my day with a 25- to 35-gram protein drink. When I am busy, it is easier to grab a protein drink, and I actually enjoy them. The answer to your question will be crystal clear to you at about six weeks after your surgery, and you will be very thankful for Inspire and Believe!

I had RNY surgery three years ago. I lost 123 pounds but have since gained back 65 pounds. I can eat anything and sugar doesn't make me sick. I am so upset that I have gained weight, I don't have anywhere else to turn, and don't know what to do.

I actually get this question quite often, so take some negative comfort in the fact that you are not alone. When you have this surgery you not only have to change your life, but the changes have to be permanent or you might not be able to keep the weight off. It isn't easy; in fact it's very difficult. The good news is that your surgery is still intact; you just have to learn how to use your limited stomach size to reduce your intake and control your total calories. You have effectively learned to eat *around* your surgery, and by making bad food choices, you are now taking in more calories than you are able to burn. You have to flip that switch in your head and first choose the protein so that you get full faster, then add nutritious vegetables, and if you have any room (which you won't, but negotiating with yourself is a good way to fool yourself) you can have a bite of a useless carb if you must.

If I make good food choices, I am able to eat about 4 ounces of rotisserie chicken and a half cup of finely chopped salad. If I didn't choose wisely I could probably eat a scoop of macaroni and cheese, a couple of bites of chicken, and half a biscuit. The total calories are not the only problem, but the *bad choice* meal will create additional hunger. Carbs are very quickly converted into glucose, and the body must release insulin to reduce the blood sugar levels. The insulin release will actually bring down the levels to below normal and create that hollow hunger. The meal of chicken and salad keeps me satisfied for hours. Even more important is that with the higher-protein meal, I retain control, and later on if I choose to I can have a sugar-free pudding cup. With the high-carb meal I would be hungry and would start looking for more food to satisfy the need to eat, and I would likely eat more carbs, creating even more hunger. I would have lost control by making the wrong food choices.

I recommend that you go back to the basics that helped you lose 123 pounds in the first place. Remove the carbohydrates from your kitchen. Inform your family that there will be no sugary or unhealthy foods until you are back in control. Plan your meals in advance and do not include any fast or processed convenience foods. If you are going to make this work you are going to have to make trade-offs and stick to your meal plans. This is not like going on a diet when we weighed 300 pounds; we now have a powerful weight-loss tool that makes it relatively easy to lose.

Always eat the protein food first; this effectively limits your capacity, because protein is more filling. Follow the protein with healthy nutrient-rich vegetables, and be sure to never drink with your meals. I recommend that you track every bite of food you put in your mouth at www.FitDay.com, because accountability helps. In addition, join our online support board at BeforeAndAfterHelp.com; we have daily accountability threads where members log in their meals. You can get ideas and guidance; plus it helps to know that there are others out there who not only understand where you are, but genuinely care about helping you to change direction. If you need help, it is out there for you!

Who inspires *you*?

I am sitting here watching the sun rise over the ocean this morning, and I realize that the world inspires me. When I was almost 300 pounds I had stopped living and had started to wish my life away; I quietly waited for events to pass so I didn't have to attend them. I will never make up for all that I have missed.

People walk into my store and don't expect to see me sitting at my desk; they stop in their tracks and sometimes begin to cry. It makes me realize just how fragile we all are when we take the step to have bariatric surgery. We are putting ourselves out there, trusting others with our survival. I have never jumped out of a plane, but I would imagine that the lead-up to the final moment when you take that step out into air is similar to the feeling we have as we are wheeled down to the operating room. Our minds run through the checklist of what to expect: Should we have gone on one more diet? Do we have the right protein for when we get home? What is our family going to eat when we're sipping broth? Are we doing the right thing? People either find my book or stumble across our website and discover that they are not the only one out there who has all the crazy thoughts flooding their mind. I am humbled by the fact that my story gives people a lifeline so that they don't feel as if they are going it alone. People tell me that I inspire them; but these are the very people who motivate me to continue to pay forward my good fortune in how this has all turned out. This surgery is rough, but you don't have to blaze your own trail. I am humbled that I am able to inspire others, but the reward is in how many people I meet who in turn inspire me!

This surgery gives people back their life, and that is what truly inspires me.

protein, carbohydrates, and sugar after weight-loss surgery

Protein

Protein is critical for repairing and replacing cell tissue as well as building new muscle. When we have major surgery such as the RNY gastric bypass procedure, protein is necessary so tissues can heal. Immediately after RNY surgery, it is nearly impossible for us to ingest adequate protein through foods alone, which is why many surgeons recommend that patients consume protein supplements via shakes. It is good nutrition for us to be able to rely on a daily protein supplement of 25 to 50 grams and add to it with high-protein, low-fat, and lower-carbohydrate foods.

How do you determine the right amount of protein for yourself? An active person needs around 1.25 grams of protein per kilogram of ideal body weight (1 kilogram equals 2.2 pounds, so divide your goal weight by 2.2). We use a person's ideal body weight to calculate protein targets because fat tissue does not need protein. Therefore a person currently weighing 247 pounds who exercises and has an ideal body weight of 145 would need 82 grams of protein daily to maintain muscle mass and good health (145 pounds divided by 2.2 pounds per kilograms then multiplied by 1.25 grams per kilogram). A person currently weighing 341 pounds with an ideal body weight of 185 would need 105 grams of protein daily to maintain muscle mass and good health (185 pounds divided by 2.2 pounds per kilogram then multi-plied by 1.25 grams per kilogram).

Note that these figures are the recommended grams of protein needed for good nutrition and to keep muscles intact. We want to lose fat, not muscle. Our vital organs are made of muscle and need protein to function efficiently. So when we talk about 65 to 100 grams of protein a day, this is not a high-protein diet, it is minimum fulfill-ment of our basic protein needs. Too little protein is a serious concern as it additionally raises the incidence of osteoporosis, which is why ap-propriate calcium supplements are also an important part of our diet.

Not only does adequate protein fend off muscle loss, but it can also speed up our fat-burning processes. Protein has the highest thermal effect of any food. This means that protein foods speed up your me-tabolism because your body has to work harder to digest, process, and use this nutrient compared to fat or carbohydrate. Use solid protein such as fish or meats as the main part of each of your three daily meals. Proteins take longer to digest and they are absorbed more slowly by your body, giving you a longer-lasting, steady source of energy.

Just as important to losing weight is the very important inhibitory effect protein has on the craving for more food. Protein is more filling and therefore we are satisfied more quickly and for a longer period with a protein meal than we would be with a high-carbohydrate meal.

Be proactive, be accountable for your health, and make sure you are getting enough protein! Grab a protein bar or a slice of turkey breast instead of a cracker or high-carb snack. Eat the protein on your plate before you even think of touching the carbohydrate.

Protein Foods Serving size	grams of protein	grams of carbohydrate
½ cup low-fat yogurt	6.5	8
½ cup 2% low-fat milk	4.0	6
½ cup 2% low-fat cottage cheese	16.0	5

before

Protein Foods Serving size	grams of protein	grams of carbohydrate
½ cup part-skim ricotta	14.0	6
1 ounce provolone cheese	7.0	0.5
1 ounce mozzarella cheese	8.0	0.8
2 ounces sliced deli ham	14.5	0
2 ounces sliced deli turkey	13.0	0
3 ounces lean ground beef, grilled	22.0	0
3 ounces beef sirloin, grilled	26.0	0
3 ounces roasted chicken, dark	22.0	0
3 ounces roasted chicken, white	26.0	0
3 ounces roasted turkey, dark	24.0	0
3 ounces roasted turkey, white	25.0	0
½ cup chicken salad	18.0	1
3 ounces broiled sole	21.0	0
3 ounces grilled tuna	23.0	0
3 ounces broiled halibut	23.0	0
3 ounces broiled red snapper	22.0	0
3 ounces broiled scallops, sautéed	18.0	2
3 ounces shrimp, peeled, steamed	21.0	1
3 ounces water-pack tuna	22.0	0
1 large egg	7.0	0.5
¼ cup almonds	7.0	7
2 tablespoons peanut butter	8.5	6

Carbohydrates

Carbohydrates are easily and readily absorbed by the body for immediate energy. When you eat a carbohydrate-loaded food, it is quickly metabolized, driving up blood sugar levels. Your body immediately responds by releasing insulin to send your blood sugar back down.

This is why a slab of warm bread, muffins, or a high-sugar food gives you a quick energy burst that soon gives way to a sluggish and tired feeling. This cycle of blood sugar highs and lows creates highs and lows of hunger. Even though you have just eaten a carbohydrate snack of crackers and are full, you are quickly hungry again because there is little lasting satisfaction in this quick fix. In addition, instead of drawing on stored fat reserves for your energy, your body burned the food you just consumed.

When you burn more calories than you consume, your body must draw on reserves to keep you going. According to acknowledged medical principles, when you cut back your intake of carbohydrates, your body converts from the metabolic process of burning carbohydrate to burning your stored fat as its primary energy source. The stored fat easily metabolizes into the components that supply energy for the body's cells, resulting in weight loss. Many of the top bariatric surgeons recommend that those of us who have RNY gastric bypass surgery consume less than 25 grams of carbohydrate per day to push our body to burn this warehoused fat for energy.

In the first few days at home after our RNY surgery, it is acceptable to have a few of the higher-carbohydrate foods as our first foods, so that we get used to eating again. A little potato soup or a few bites of bean puree or hummus are higher in carbohydrates but are safe, soft foods that will not burden our swollen stomach and intestines. We really cannot ingest enough of these higher-carbohydrate foods at this point to hurt us. By the time we start to feel better, we become aware of protein and can redirect our diets.

Our surgeons and nutritionists all tell us to eat protein first, but as we heal and get back into cooking for our families, preparing meals for ourselves, and eating in restaurants, we need to know how to choose foods that will keep carbohydrate consumption to a minimum. Generally speaking, any food that comes from a growing plant or is processed from a product grown in the ground is a carbohydrate. Milk and dairy products are also included because they contain lactose ("milk sugar"). We are looking for the highest protein, vitamins, and minerals for the lowest amount of carbs. Fortunately, some of the most nutritious vegetables and fruits have the lowest carbohydrate counts. I have included a basic list of lower-carb vegetables. Usually the more watery or acidic vegetables are lower in carbs than the starchier or sweeter vegetables. If you can choose either a small dish of zucchini or half a baked potato, the zucchini is a much better choice as it provides fiber, vitamins, and other nutrients, but very few carbohydrates. The potato provides too few nutrients to warrant using up your entire daily carbohydrate budget. A quarter-cup portion of spinach sautéed with garlic is packed with nutrients, whereas an equal amount of pasta salad provides nothing of consequence but unwanted carbohydrates. A few cubes of tomato tossed with shredded romaine are a much better choice than a small dish of corn in terms of nutrition. Sautéed sliced asparagus has fiber and a high nutritional value when compared to a scoop of rice or a small dinner roll. Look at your 25 grams of daily carbohydrates as an allowance and make good choices to spend your carbohydrate grams wisely, choosing vegetables and fruits that provide the most nutrients in combination with the fewest grams of carbohydrate. Eating after RNY gastric bypass surgery is all about making good choices. Have a bite of the baked potato or pasta salad if you need to satisfy your taste for it, but be aware of the trade-off you are making and have a few bites of the more nutritious selection as well.

Vegetable Carbohydrate Counts

		grams of carbohydrate
Arugula	½ cup baby leaves, raw	0.4
Romaine	½ cup shredded, raw	0.6
Mushrooms	¼ cup sliced, raw	0.7
Bok Choy	¼ cup sliced, cooked	0.7

Cucumber	¼ cup sliced, raw	0.7
Cabbage	¼ cup shredded, raw	0.8
Radishes	¼ cup sliced, raw	1.0
Asparagus	2 medium spears, cooked	1.2
Zucchini	¼ cup sliced, cooked	1.3
Cauliflower	¼ cup chopped, cooked	1.5
Spinach	¼ cup chopped, cooked	1.6
Fennel	¼ cup sliced, cooked	1.6
Eggplant	¼ cup diced, cooked	1.6
Swiss Chard	¼ cup sliced, cooked	1.8
Tomato	¼ cup diced, raw or canned	1.8
Broccoli	¼ cup chopped, cooked	1.9
Green Beans	¼ cup sliced, cooked	2.3
Collard Greens	¼ cup chopped, cooked	2.3
Green Pepper	¼ cup diced, raw	2.4
Avocado	¼ small Hass variety	3.2
Onion	¼ cup chopped, raw	3.2
Artichoke Hearts	¼ cup sliced, canned	4.1
Carrots	¼ cup sliced, cooked	4.1
Peas	¼ cup cooked	5.0
Brussels Sprouts	4 small whole	7.8
Corn	¼ cup kernels, cooked	10.6
Sweet Potato	½ small, roasted	13.9
Potato	½ small, baked	25.4

Fruit Carbohydrate Counts

		grams of carbohydrate
Strawberries	½ cup sliced, fresh	2.9
Raspberries	½ cup whole, fresh	3.5
Plum	½ small 2-inch fruit	4.2
Peach	½ small 2½-inch fruit	4.3

		grams of carbohydrate
Watermelon	½ cup small cubes	5.1
Blueberries	¼ cup whole, fresh	5.1
Orange	¼ cup chopped sections	5.3
Kiwi	½ whole fruit	5.6
Cherries	¼ cup pitted, fresh	6.0
Cantaloupe	½ cup small cubes	6.6
Honeydew	½ cup small cubes	7.8
Nectarine	½ small 2½-inch fruit	8.0
Apple	½ small 2½-inch fruit	9.5
Pineapple	½ cup cubes, fresh/canned in juice	9.6
Pear, fresh	½ small	10.7
Pear, canned	½ cup, diced, no sugar added	14.2
Banana	½ cup, sliced	15.8
Grapes	½ cup seedless, white or red	15.8
Banana	1 small (6–7 inch), whole	23.0

Sugar and Dumping Syndrome

If people who have had RNY gastric bypass surgery eat foods with high levels of sugar or fat, they risk experiencing the wrath of "dumping syndrome." When we ingest a high volume of sugar or fat, our body attempts to dilute the food by drawing large amounts of liquid into the intestine from the blood. This causes a rapid drop in blood pressure and a significant rise in blood sugar, which in turn prods the pancreas to release insulin. This insulin release is so strong that it sends the now-high blood sugar levels plummeting, causing a combination of intense nausea, profuse sweating, faintness, weakness, severe and immediate intestinal cramping, and then explosive diarrhea. Most people who have experienced it say it is so awful that they will do anything they can to avoid having it happen again. I experienced a mild dumping episode only once and it was one of the most unpleasant physical experiences I have ever had.

People who have had RNY gastric bypass surgery must always monitor their sugar intake. Be proactive and become a relentless label reader, since sugar is found in products that you would never suspect. There are excellent sugar-free products to satisfy an occasional desire for something sweet, so we don't need to sabotage our success by pushing the envelope and discovering our dumping level. I would rather not know exactly how much sugar triggers my mechanism; the fear of dumping keeps me from eating a hunk of layer cake. Dumping provides strong negative feedback and therefore limits the undesirable behavior. A weight-loss-surgery friend of mine who is now at her goal weight says, "Dumping is like having a personal food cop with you at all times so you can't hide in your closet and eat like you did pre-op." Limit your sugar intake to 5 to 8 grams at one time, at the end of a meal, to err on the side of caution. It is believed that dumping occurs when the sugar load is greater than 15 grams at one time, but tolerance levels can and will vary. Dumping can also occur when we eat too much of any food, but it is most common with sugar and fat.

If we make good choices a part of our lives now, we will have long-term success with our weight loss. If we make bad choices now while we are severely limited in our stomach capacity, what choices will we make when we can eat larger portions in two years? If you are regularly eating 125 grams of carbohydrate in a day and have discovered that you do not "dump" on sugar at three months post-op, what will you be eating at 18 months post-op? If we change our relationship with food now, it will be second nature to us in the future, and we will never have to diet again.

food stages and early meal plans

You are home from the hospital and resting uncomfortably on the sofa. All the notes you took as a pre-op are written in Greek, and you don't remember what you are supposed to eat.

The surgical modifications made to your body require *permanent* changes in eating habits from the start and must be closely adhered to in order to not injure yourself and later to maximize the opportunity for weight loss. Post-surgery dietary guidelines can vary greatly by bariatric surgeon; you will hear of other patients who have been given different rules following their weight-loss surgery. It is important that you follow *your* surgeon's recommended time line. This information is not intended to replace that which your center has given you but to clarify and give you some practical real life ideas to get through this initial learning curve of uncertainty.

You are not hungry; you just think you are. Do not allow imaginary head hunger to advance your diet ahead of schedule. When you feel as if you want to eat, have a sugar-free ice pop or some flavored water, or take a walk, even if only to the mailbox.

Use small plates and bowls; we work to finish what is on our plate and serve ourselves portions based on our plate size. Put your fork down on the table between bites. Try not to gulp air with your food. Don't use a straw as air is swallowed along with the liquid and can be uncomfortable.

A dish of macaroni and cheese may *seem* like a soft food to you, but it is not a good food choice. Do not eat breads, pasta, or rice as these foods are gummy and can create great discomfort and vomiting.

This is your fresh start to change your relationship with food; the absolute line in the sand.

Take your vitamins immediately prior to a small meal of yogurt, a bite of cheese, or sugar-free pudding to lessen the likelihood of nausea. Do not take vitamins on an empty stomach as they often cause stomach upset. If your vitamins are making you sick, wait and start taking them in a later stage when you are able to have more food in the pouch.

Remember that if at *any* time you are repeatedly vomiting liquids or water, or if simply drinking water or eating the right foods is painful, call your doctor.

Clear Liquids

In the first stage after surgery we are restricted to clear liquids, generally any fluid you can see through. Doctors require anywhere from a few days to a week of clear fluids after surgery. They are easy to digest and do not leave much residue in the stomach and intestines while maintaining vital body fluids, salts, and minerals.

It is not uncommon to be rehospitalized due to dehydration, so it is important to be aware of fluid intake. Take small drinks of liquid every few minutes and increase as tolerated so you are drinking at least two quarts (64 ounces) of fluid a day. You should have a sports bottle near you at all times and sip almost continuously.

Warm drinks are soothing as the heat relaxes the muscles and tissues of the pouch. There are clear proteins (listed below) that will help your body to heal more rapidly. If any drink tastes too sweet, add more water, or add crushed ice to dilute it to your taste.

> **Water**
> **Crystal Light—use two to three times more water than directed, as
> it will taste much too sweet**

Sugar-free Jell-O

Ocean Spray Diet Cranberry or Diet Blueberry Pomegranate

Noncarbonated, sugar-free, zero-calorie fruit waters

Diet Snapple

Herbal tea—a mug of warm Celestial Seasonings tea is very soothing

Broth or bouillon—chicken or beef

Sugar-free Popsicles

Full Liquids

Full liquids include those that are somewhat pourable and smooth. Begin to use protein drinks to give your body the building materials needed to heal from the trauma of the surgery.

The goal in this phase is to introduce more calories into your diet and ready your surgically altered stomach and intestines for your first food. Doctors vary in their requirements for length of time in this food stage; some as little as a day, others as long as a month. Stay with your surgeon's prescribed time line.

During this phase, food may continue to have an off taste, and some foods, usually dairy products, will cause stomach rumbling and gas. Focus on fluids first and get plenty of rest—it gets better every day!

Do not drink for thirty minutes to one hour after meals to avoid washing the slightly thickened foods through the pouch. You may not think that this scheduling has a point, but it will become clearer to you in subsequent phases. Learning not to drink either with or after meals will be extremely important throughout your post-operative life.

The following items can be added to the list of clear liquids that are already in your pantry:

Protein shakes, drinks, and soups—I've worked with specialists and food scientists to develop our own line of protein products. Inspire whey protein isolate drink mixes and soup mixes

contain the correct nutrition for bariatric post-ops, but it's just as important that they taste great, because we're a picky group of people. All protein products available on BariatricEating .com are preselected for our dietary guidelines and good taste. Don't be fooled by popular TV brands of "weight-loss" protein, as they contain very little protein per serving; it's also the lowest-quality protein type, known as whey concentrate. Whey protein concentrate contains impurities and lactose and is not as efficiently absorbed. Whey protein isolate (WPI) is the best protein for bariatric post-op patients. Always read the labels of products you buy and pay attention to sugar and carb content. Some of these brands contain alarming amounts of sugar. A good rule of thumb is for a serving of protein to contain 20 to 25 grams of protein, about 120 calories, and 5 to 10 grams of carbohydrate, of which fewer than 5 grams should be sugar.

Plain yogurt or light yogurt that does not contain added sugar or fruit pieces—check the list of ingredients—if it says fructose, sugar, honey, evaporated cane juice, or high-fructose corn syrup, it has added sugar. Notice that even plain yogurt will show grams of sugar on the "Nutrition Facts" label, as yogurt contains naturally occurring sugar called lactose; however, this is not added sugar. It is always best to buy plain or Greek yogurt and add a little no-added-sugar strained baby food fruit, a fork-mashed banana, or sugar-free seedless preserves to flavor and sweeten. The low-carb food-starch-thickened products that are out there are not really yogurt; while they may be low in carbs, they provide little nutrition and do not give you all the wonderful benefits of yogurt.

Skim milk

Unsweetened almond milk—refrigerated brands in the dairy section taste better than shelf-stable brands

Silk Light Vanilla—this soy milk has great vanilla flavor and

before

is sweetened with all-natural, zero-calorie stevia, with 70 calories and 6 grams protein per serving. It's great tasting, and lactose and dairy free. The chocolate flavor is too high in sugar, so again, make sure you read labels and not assume because one flavor is low in sugar that all are.

Jell-O sugar-free pudding—ready-made or use instant prepared with skim milk (instant pudding does not thicken using soy or almond milk)

Vanilla Egg Custard (page 143)

Creamed soups (this does not mean soups with cream but refers to texture)—puree Progresso Lentil, Hearty Black Bean, or Minestrone soup, or Amy's Organic Light in Sodium Chunky Tomato Bisque, in a blender until smooth. After heating, blend in a small amount of Pure Unflavored Whey Protein Isolate to add protein.

Very thin potato "soup" made by blending Idahoan Mashed Potatoes flakes into homemade or low-sodium chicken broth. Stick with the original or plain potato rather than any of the flavors. I chose this brand because it contains 100 percent natural potato flakes and comes in small envelopes to use by the spoonful.

Tomato juice or V8—warmed or chilled

The following are examples of how to use allowed foods to create meals. Start off with ¼ cup as a guide, and understand that you may not feel full with these consistencies, as they are soft and semi-liquid. Never force food or liquid—if you feel full, stop.

Breakfast

¼ cup Cream of Wheat or Cream of Rice prepared with skim milk and thinned out to a pourable texture with a little Believe Vanilla Creme Brulee Protein Drink

Midmorning planned protein and fluid break

> **Inspire Hot Chocolate with Marshmallows whey protein isolate
> drink mix made with hot water**

Lunch

> **¼ cup Dannon or Fage Total 0% Greek yogurt blended with a
> spoonful of Inspire Peanut Butter Cookie whey protein isolate
> drink mix**

Midafternoon planned protein and fluid break

> **½ cup V8 Vegetable Juice**

Supper

> **Inspire Mexican Taco Soup whey protein isolate mix**

Other breakfast choices

> **½ Vanilla Egg Custard (page 143)**
> **½ Jell-O sugar-free pudding cup blended with a teaspoon of
> Inspire Peanut Butter Fudge whey protein isolate
> drink mix**
> **1 scoop Inspire Dutch Chocolate Cake whey protein isolate drink
> mix made with water**
> **1 scoop Inspire Summer Melon whey protein isolate drink mix
> made with water**
> **Inspire Hot Chocolate with Marshmallows whey protein isolate
> drink mix made using hot water**
> **Believe Coconut Protein Energy Drink**

Other lunch or supper choices

> **Potato soup—heat 1 cup Swanson Natural Goodness Chicken
> Broth, then whisk in 2 tablespoons Idahoan Original potato
> flakes to create a thin, smooth soup. To make this even better,
> whisk in 1 teaspoon grated Parmesan and 1 tablespoon Pure
> Unflavored Whey Protein Isolate.**
>
> **Inspire Mexican Taco Soup whey protein isolate mix**
>
> **Inspire Lasagna Soup whey protein isolate mix**
>
> **Inspire Hot Chocolate with Marshmallows whey protein isolate
> drink mix made using hot water**
>
> **Believe Coconut Protein Energy Drink**

Supplement choices for midmorning and midafternoon

> **1 bottle Believe Vanilla Creme Brulee or Coconut Protein Energy
> Drink**
>
> **1 scoop Inspire whey protein isolate drink mix blended with water
> or almond or soy milk in a shaker cup**
>
> **1 cup Crystal Light Lemonade blended with 1 teaspoon Pure
> Unflavored Whey Protein Isolate**
>
> **Inspire Hot Chocolate with Marshmallows whey protein isolate
> drink mix made using hot water**

Purees and Soft Foods

Your surgeon will indicate when it is time for you to advance to the
puree and then soft diet. While it is frustrating to be *held back* in these
special phases, advancing too rapidly into foods that are too dense or
solid may put pressure on the staple line, causing breakage or leaking,
and can cause vomiting or even result in foods getting stuck, so be patient and do not push the limits of this stage. If at any time you find that

you are not doing well with these foods or experience vomiting, go back to the full liquid phase—remain for a day, then slowly advance again.

Initially all foods are pureed and should be soft and loose; the consistency of applesauce is a good reference for texture for this phase. You will slowly progress to foods that can be finely mashed with a fork or chewed to a soft moist mouthful. There is a blurred line between purees and soft foods, as they are basically the same foods in slightly different states.

In this stage protein will begin to be an *essential* part of your diet. Protein heals wounds, repairs skin and muscle, creates fullness, or *satiety*, and will minimize hair loss and promote regrowth. Each meal and snack should contain a good source of protein.

You should eat three small meals per day plus protein supplements midmorning and midafternoon in order to get in adequate nutrition. Some surgeons call this *five small meals*. The puree diet includes the foods you have already been using plus very soft foods such as the following:

Eggs
Low-fat cheese, mozzarella sticks, sliced deli cheese such as Swiss or Muenster
Low-fat cottage cheese
Part-skim ricotta cheese
Small amounts of mashed banana for flavoring
No Sugar Added Applesauce or Cinammon Applesauce (page 142)
Pureed canned beans such as pinto or black beans
Tender mild white fish filets—tilapia, sole, flounder, cod
Shrimp and crab (not imitation crab, which may contain sugar)

Hint: a small food processor produces a finely ground texture, while a blender creates a dense paste that is often sticky and not easy to eat.

The following are examples of meals using foods that are allowed during the puree stage, and then in a more textured state in the soft food stage. I still eat these simply prepared *meals* as a long-term post-op as they are good food choices for the rest of our lives; high in protein, low in carbohydrates, easy to eat, and delicious!

Breakfast—choose one

> **A softly scrambled egg omelet with a thin slice of low-fat cheese. (In the soft food stage add a spoonful of your favorite salsa or prepared spaghetti sauce. Read labels; choose brands that do not have sugar or high-fructose corn syrup in the ingredient list.)**
>
> **¼ cup plain yogurt blended with 1 teaspoon Inspire Pistachio whey protein isolate drink mix (or Inspire Summer Melon, or Natural Vanilla Very Berry, or Dutch Chocolate Cake, with a few slices of banana—get creative)**
>
> **¼ cup part-skim milk ricotta blended with your favorite flavor of Inspire whey protein isolate drink mix**
>
> **¼ cup low-fat cottage cheese and 2 tablespoons unsweetened applesauce sprinkled with Splenda and cinnamon**
>
> **A frosty blended protein shake made with a dollop of yogurt, a scoop of Inspire Natural Vanilla Very Berry, a few frozen berries, ¼ cup almond milk, and 5 or 6 ice cubes. Pulse in the blender until silky smooth.**
>
> **A ready-to-drink (RTD) protein drink such as OhYeah! Strawberry and Creme protein minis—8-ounce bottles that contain 18 grams of protein and taste like the strawberry powder we used to add to milk when we were kids. Believe protein energy drink flavors are also excellent choices that contain 500 mg of calcium and an over-the-top supply of B vitamins.**

Lunch and supper—choose one for each meal

> **Pouch or canned tuna finely mashed with a small amount of light mayonnaise and low-fat Newman's Own salad dressing for flavoring.**
>
> **Part-skim ricotta cheese with a spoonful of prepared spaghetti sauce and shredded mozzarella, warmed in microwave. (Read labels; Classico, Barilla, and Gia Russa are brands that do not have sugar or high-fructose corn syrup in their ingredient list.)**
>
> **A good quality canned soup such as Progresso black bean or lentil pulsed in the blender or food processor—do *not* choose brands or flavors that have more than 5 grams of sugar or contain noodles or rice. (Tomato soup has too much sugar; read the label.)**
>
> **Tilapia fish filet, poached in tomato juice or chicken broth, finely mashed with some of the cooking liquid.**
>
> **A scrambled egg whisked into a cup of simmering broth.**
>
> **An egg poached or simmered in prepared spaghetti sauce (page 154).**
>
> **Pinto Bean Dip (page 135)—dips, spreads, and soups are prepared smooth for the puree stage and chunkier for the soft food stage.**
>
> **Shrimp Salad Spread (page 136).**
>
> **Creamy Black Bean Soup (page 130).**
>
> **Creamy Tuscan Bean Soup (page 132).**

After a transitional period where you are doing well with the softer pureed foods and are getting more comfortable with eating again, you can slowly begin to add soft foods and prepare the recipes from the next chapter. There is only a fine line between these stages, and if at any time you don't feel well in your choices, drop back to full liquids and the softer purees until you can move forward again. An example of a soft food would be a fish filet simmered in some mild salsa or prepared spaghetti sauce rather than broth or tomato juice; turkey chili; boneless chicken thigh pieces simmered in seasoned broth until they can be mashed; or a finely chopped ham and cheese one-egg omelet. Soft meals contain the same foods but with slightly more texture. You will still rely on the purees as they will always be easy to eat.

Many programs tell patients that after a few weeks of soft foods they can incorporate *regular foods* into our diets, and this isn't always interpreted correctly. After eleven years, I still pay attention to food textures; baked chicken breast, half of a sandwich, or grilled pork chop will be too dry and dense and will cause me to throw up and feel sick for hours. Do not take the term "regular or normal foods" literally as we will *always* need to pay attention to not only the nutrition but also the moisture and consistency of the foods we select.

protein drinks

For the first weeks after surgery, the stomach pouch and the *stoma*, or opening into the intestine, are swollen and small. I started drinking protein shakes within days of returning home from the hospital and have had one or more a day ever since. The cold frostiness was soothing to my stomach and it took the place of my morning coffee while I read my e-mail. There are many of us who have had the surgery, tried one sip of one protein shake, decided we did not like the smell or taste, and declined further protein supplements.

After going through such an extreme surgical procedure to regain life and good health, it should go without saying that we need to make a serious commitment to using protein supplements for as long we need them. It will be a long time before you are able to eat enough protein via food; in fact it is likely you may *never* be able to meet your protein requirements through food alone, and therefore must make up the difference using protein supplements. It is fast and risk-free to grab a protein drink, and with the brands I use, it is enjoyable.

When I had my surgery several years ago the protein shake choices were limited to bad chocolate, bad strawberry, and vanilla. I discovered that vanilla made a good base for thick frosty blender shakes, and with the addition of a few simple ingredients I could make it taste like a Dairy Queen Blizzard. I am proud to say that people who hated protein shakes loved them once they followed my suggestions.

I rarely make blender drinks these days as protein formulas have changed greatly over even the last three years and the new proteins literally melt into water and need minimal blending. I now prefer thin textured drinks, but those thick creamy frozen concoctions I ate with a spoon when I first started this journey are still the best thing going for a new post-op.

Each time we read a muscle magazine or go to the gym, Ty and I notice new products; and we're quick to taste every protein drink and bar that we find. I share the information on particular products because I use them myself and find they make my life easier. It was a chore to have to assemble so many products from so many different sources for my personal use. I knew early on that for my own health I would need to develop a long-term love of protein supplements and keep in touch with the latest and best products—so we developed our website, www.BariatricEating.com.

The greatest reward for the work we've put into creating our bariatric business has been the overwhelming positive response by the bariatric surgeons and their staff who wholeheartedly recommend our products, website, book, and message board. They recognize that anything that makes life easier, tastier, and healthier for their patients will increase compliance. If you can easily find the best products, you will more closely adhere to their program and change your life!

No matter what brands you decide taste best to your palate, make sure your protein is a very low carbohydrate formula with minimal sugar; there are versions for weight gain and bodybuilding that are high in carbs and sugar and are not for bariatric use. Read the labels carefully before you choose if you go it on your own using the nutrition center route.

Most bariatric programs require that we use protein drinks until we are able to take in at least 75 grams of protein per day via our food. We must use these drinks to make up the difference between what we need and what we can comfortably eat. For many, this means that protein drinks will be a part of our lives for anywhere from a few months to a lifetime, while others rely on protein drinks by choice as a grab-and-go solution to skipping a meal. Even though it has been more than eleven years since my surgery, I often use a protein drink instead of a meal as a reliable source of sustenance. When I travel and don't have a regular schedule, it's safer for me to have a protein drink in my hotel room so I don't have to worry about a situation in which my blood sugar levels dip too low. When traveling on business or with friends, others may decide to delay a meal or have a large breakfast and forgo lunch, so I carry protein powder, a bottled drink, or a protein bar and packets of nuts with me in order to keep a somewhat regular independent schedule. One of the most important long-term lessons I've learned is to be prepared and able to take care of my own food needs.

You've probably had a negative first experience with supermarket protein drinks. Protein drinks are not a punishment when you know how to make them—it just takes a little time and persistence to learn how to work with them. I'm always happy to hear stories of your gym-bound sons, daughters, and spouses sneaking your protein shakes once they taste the delicious concoctions you've created from your bags, canisters, and bottles of powders! I've been doing this so long that I can make any protein drinkable with a few additions, but it's a lot easier to start with a great-tasting base.

Rather than having to constantly find new bodybuilder products that work for our specific medical needs, I've taken matters into my own hands to develop brands and flavors of protein drinks for us under my SML label. My protein drinks taste great and have amazing nutrition, and I can also promise that our products are absolute top quality and manufactured in clean GMP-certified facilities.

The most time-effective way to drink protein is by grabbing a ready-to-drink bottle, can, or juice box tetra pack, called an RTD. While this is the most convenient choice, it's also the most expensive, and many RTDs have a terrible aftertaste, a thick and unpleasant consistency, and problems with chunking up in the container. We carry only a few brands of RTDs in our web stores because we sample everything on the market and choose the ones that we personally like to drink. It's easy to make bad-tasting protein, and that is why there is so much of it on the market.

Believe bottled protein lattes, chai tea, and vanilla flavors are the bestselling premium drinks for bariatric post-ops or anyone who is health conscious. Each 9.5-ounce bottle contains 20 grams of protein and 500 mg of calcium, plus the coffee and chai flavors provide a huge B vitamin boost that exceeds daily requirements. The best part is the enjoyable flavor and thin, smooth texture—think of a Starbucks Frappuccino in a bottle! Italian Cappuccino is a sweetened latte with a touch of vanilla and nut. Mocha Latte is a true chocolate latte. Smooth Chai Tea is a cinnamon-spiced gingerbread cookie, and Vanilla Creme Brulee, a caramel vanilla, is the only caffeine-free flavor.

I'm a morning coffee drinker and will use a single bottle of Believe Mocha Latte in place of creamer in my first two mugs of coffee—turning my mugs of steaming hot java into two amazing protein lattes! If you're not a breakfast eater, there's no better way to take in a reliable 20 grams of protein before nine in the morning.

We have additional flavors in development, including premium Chocolate, Coconut and Mango protein drinks, and even a line of gourmet, ready-to-heat-and-eat protein soups.

Next, make protein shakes using protein powders. It's important to start with a high-quality base to make your shakes. A keg of vanilla protein that you picked up at the local warehouse club is not a bargain when you can't drink it and your hair falls out! Start with a high-quality vanilla protein isolate that does not have a strong smell or aftertaste—it will make your job as a mixologist easier, and you'll look forward to your protein shakes and smile when everyone else in your support group is complaining.

Honestly, if my surgeon had told me that I had to drink a dirt milk shake every day for the rest of my life to keep off the lost weight, I would have happily asked him, "How much dirt?" But many post-op patients are picky. Be open-minded about protein and keep trying different brands and flavors using my tips, and you'll eventually find one you love to drink. It's either that or lose your hair—you choose.

Rule number one: Avoid lumping and clumping by always adding liquid to the powder. This is a tip I learned way back in freshman chemistry, thanks to Mr. Leighton Wass. Now go back and read that again and think about it—add the liquid to the powder. If you add the powder to a shaker cup filled with liquid, you will end up with an island of floating powder and the bottom of that island will not blend; it will remain as lumps in your drink.

When people write or call us about protein shakes clumping up, it's almost always because they have it backward. Put your scoop of protein powder into the bottom of your dry shaker cup or glass and add your liquid to the powder. Then shake or stir for smooth perfection. Try it and you'll be amazed at the difference. Pass it on and you'll be a rock star in your surgeon's support group.

All protein shakes were blender drinks when I had my surgery in 2001. These days, with new processes, some powders can be blended in a shaker cup or even in a glass using a spoon.

We created Inspire to be the perfect protein drink in taste, texture, and nutrition for anyone looking for a quality protein drink for bariatric, weight-loss, fitness, or medical needs. It blends so easily that I have mixed it while sitting in the middle seat of a completely full airplane, using two small plastic cups, water, and no spoon!

Inspire whey protein isolate drink mix offers yummy flavors like Dutch Chocolate Cake, Ice Cream Sandwich, Chocolate Peanut Butter Fudge, Pistachio, Caramel Latte, Cinnamon Cappuccino, Raspberry Lemonade, Natural Vanilla Very Berry, Vanilla

Date, Pomegranate Berry, and Summer Melon. We start with clean pure unflavored Whey Protein Isolate and flavor it in the same way I would cook with real foods in my own kitchen—with real cocoa, vanilla, toasted ground nuts, ground berries, natural fruit flavors, and extracts—so that our protein drinks taste bright and flavorful!

Inspire Dutch Chocolate Cake is the best chocolate protein drink on the planet. It's not too sweet and has a deep cocoa flavor. The Inspire flavors are made to blend with small amounts of water—most people find the proper flavor is achieved by blending a single scoop with just 4 to 8 ounces of water! So a small, delicious Inspire drink contains 20 to 25 grams of the best-quality protein, yet has zero sugar, zero fat, zero carbs, and just 120 calories.

Even better news is that you can turn that single scoop of Inspire Dutch Chocolate Cake into a delicious gourmet mug of warm cocoa. In fact, several of our Inspire flavors are even better warm than they are cold. Inspire Peanut Butter Cookie tastes like a hot-from-the-oven peanut butter cookie when made into a warm drink.

If you're a coffee lover, Inspire Cinnamon Cappuccino and Caramel Latte are exceptional blended into your cup of coffee. Good-bye, Starbucks!

Early on, a warm protein drink soothes the pouch—so if you've just returned home from the hospital, try your Inspire made as a warm drink. You'll thank me!

How to turn Inspire whey protein isolate drink mix flavors into a mug of warm goodness:

1. Place a scoop of protein into a clean, dry mug.
2. Add about 2 tablespoons of tap water and use a spoon to blend it into a smooth paste. Allow to rest 30 seconds if needed.
3. Slowly add hot but *not* boiling liquid to the paste while stirring to blend.

While it may seem faster to blend it all up and microwave it, if you boil your drink once protein has been added, you'll get cooked lumps and your drink will be grainy rather than smooth.

Tips:

Use Coffee-Mate Sugar Free Liquid creamer instead of tap water in step 2

Fill your mug with about a cup (or to taste) of hot coffee instead of water

Think outside the box—Inspire Peanut Butter Cookie is out of this world as a warm drink!

For an occasional treat, add a small swirl of Land O Lakes Sugar-Free Whipped Cream to kick your warm protein drink up a notch

Pure Unflavored Whey Protein Isolate will change your post-surgical life! It completely dissolves into just a small tablespoon or two of water and can then be blended into any semi-liquid food or liquid without changing the taste or texture. Pure is the purest, most unflavored whey isolate obtainable. While other companies have no idea where their whey protein comes from or even what country, ours comes from a single source within the United States. There are other brands of unflavored whey isolate for sale, but none comes close to this superb product.

For best results, blend Pure using the method for making warm cocoa. Dissolve 1 or 2 small scoops of Pure into a bit of liquid, then blend your hot tomato soup, chicken or beef broth, chili, or bean soup into the liquefied Pure—or, on the sweet side, you can blend it into Crystal Light, Splenda-sweetened juice drinks, yogurt, or the drink of your choice. Also try blending cold V8 juice into liquid Pure—many early post-ops have a craving for salt, and this V8 protein cocktail quenches that need.

Blender Shakes

protein shake pantry ingredients

> Frozen banana pieces—cut peeled ripe bananas into 1-inch
> chunks, freeze on a plate, and store in a freezer bag
> Frozen pineapple cubes—buy frozen pineapple chunks, or divide a
> can of Dole Crushed Pineapple in natural juice into sections of a
> plastic ice cube tray—freeze, pop out, and store in a freezer bag
> Coconut, maple, peppermint, vanilla, rum, and almond extracts
> Ground cinnamon
> Peanut butter
> Ghirardelli Unsweetened Cocoa powder
> DaVinci, Artista, and Torani sugar-free syrups

Isopure Perfect Natural Vanilla is an amazing base for a flavored blender shake. While I think that Isopure's Perfect Natural Chocolate is excellent, I can make a chocolate shake by adding a tablespoon of cocoa to my vanilla, and chocolate is less flexible if you're buying only one canister. Isopure has been around for ages, and it is a top-quality company.

You can always buy cheaper protein, but it will not contain the same compounds as a quality product such as Inspire or Isopure. In addition, cheaper protein, called protein concentrate, contains less bioavailable protein, meaning less gets used by your body. The most obvious difference is that cheap doesn't taste good—and if you don't drink it, it wasn't a good deal after all. The best protein drink is the one that you look forward to drinking. This is why our Inspire flavors are so popular—the flavors are excellent.

Think about protein drinks in terms of recipe flavors. If you like peach cobbler, understand that to make a real peach cobbler, we would use peaches, butter, flour, sugar, and cinnamon, and top it with a scoop of vanilla ice cream. To make a peach cobbler protein smoothie, we would use Isopure Perfect Natural Vanilla, Splenda-sweetened peaches, cinnamon, a drop of vanilla, Greek yogurt, and ice.

To bake brownies in the kitchen, we would use cocoa, vanilla, and nuts—so for a chocolate brownie shake, we would use Isopure Perfect Natural Vanilla, cocoa powder, Splenda, a few almonds or walnuts, and ice.

Technique is important as well. If you put it all in the blender and flip on the switch, you'll quickly have a blender full of fluffy foam that is difficult to drink. Instead, toggle the switch on the blender and pulse your drink in two-second on/offs, and in a minute you'll have a thick, smooth, frosty shake, similar to what you'd have gotten at McDonald's in your previous life. Proportion is important as well—do not use a lot of liquid; we want a small, drinkable shake, not an entire 48-ounce blender full.

Protein drinks are designed to blend smoothly with water these days. Milk can be a bone-healthy addition later in post-op life, but don't use it in your shakes. Early on, milk will give you a lot of gas—as bariatric surgery creates lactose intolerance that lasts a lifetime for some—plus the carbs and calories are just wasted, as shakes taste great when made with water and flavorings.

In the old days, the more fattening the better when making a milk shake, but these days we go for lots of flavor and protein, with as few carbohydrates and calories as possible. I do notice while reading posts on our message board that some people have added an entire banana to their protein shake, but a small banana can contain 30 carbs, and that much natural sugar can and will often make us sick. Go with a small piece of banana to flavor a shake—cut a whole banana into 1-inch pieces, pop them into a Ziploc bag, and pull them out one at a time for your shakes.

the perfect strawberry yogurt
protein smoothie

½ cup Blue Diamond Original Almond Breeze milk

1 scoop Pure Unflavored Whey Protein Isolate powder

½ cup plain Greek yogurt

1 heaping tablespoon Smucker's Sugar Free Strawberry Preserves

Splenda to taste

6 frozen strawberries

¼ teaspoon vanilla extract

1½ cups ice cubes

peach cobbler smoothie

4 slices Splenda-sweetened canned peaches

1 scoop Isopure Perfect Natural Vanilla protein powder

¼ teaspoon ground cinnamon

½ cup Greek yogurt

1 drop almond extract

¼ cup water

1 cup ice cubes

vermont banana protein smoothie

1 scoop Isopure Perfect Natural Vanilla protein powder

1 frozen banana chunk

½ teaspoon maple extract

½ cup water

1 cup ice cubes

piña colada smoothie

1 scoop Isopure Perfect Natural Vanilla protein powder
½ cup plain yogurt
2 packets Splenda
2 frozen pineapple cubes
½ teaspoon coconut extract
1 drop rum extract
½ cup water
1 cup ice cubes

elvis's favorite smoothie

1 scoop Inspire Peanut Butter Cookie whey protein isolate
    drink mix
One 2-inch chunk ripe banana or 1 drop banana extract
½ cup skim milk
1 cup ice cubes

berry yogurt smoothie

½ cup frozen blueberries, raspberries, or blackberries
1 scoop Isopure Perfect Natural Vanilla protein powder
½ cup Greek yogurt
¼ cup water
1 cup ice cubes

mexican chocolate smoothie

1 scoop Inspire Dutch Chocolate Cake whey protein isolate
    drink mix
1 teaspoon cocoa powder

2 packets Splenda

½ teaspoon almond extract

¼ teaspoon ground cinnamon

½ cup water

1 cup ice cubes

frozen cappuccino

1 scoop Inspire Caramel Latte whey protein isolate drink mix

1 cup cold strong coffee

¼ teaspoon ground cinnamon

1 cup ice cubes

chocolate-covered cherry smoothie

1 scoop Inspire Dutch Chocolate Cake whey protein isolate
    drink mix

5 frozen cherries

¼ teaspoon almond extract

½ cup water

1 cup ice cubes

Life after bariatric surgery is what you make of it. It's going to be a smoother ride if you are positive and happy about all the wonderful flavors you can have while you use protein drinks to *fuel* your weight loss, rather than living in sadness, mourning the flavors you believe you are losing. We lose nothing after surgery but our morbid obesity—while we gain self-confidence, health, and life.

soups, purees, and other soft foods

The first real foods eaten after returning home from the hospital are liquids and purees, followed by soft foods. Surgeons' opinions as to how long we should eat in each category vary, but even a week seems an eternity unless you've planned ahead for some variety. It was easier right from the start to make foods that my whole family could enjoy, instead of preparing separate meals, and I decided that soups would be easiest. When you have a soothing cup of black bean soup to sip, you won't be pressing yourself to move on to the next stage. I made a pot of potato soup and served it to my husband with a salad and crusty loaf of French bread my first week home after surgery. For the first two to three weeks we don't need to be as concerned with carbohydrate counts due to the small amounts we are consuming, so don't let the potato soup worry you. I was happy just sipping my delicious soup, and he marveled that I was eating with him 10 days after gastric bypass surgery. I served small ramekins of sugar-free vanilla pudding for dessert with a dollop of Splenda-sweetened whipped cream. It was a major victory for me both physically and spiritually.

A large egg has 7 grams of protein and less than 1 gram of carbohydrate. For the first six months after my surgery, I couldn't stand the texture of hard-cooked egg, so I used eggs in custards, tarts, and omelets to sneak in a few extra grams of soft protein. I enjoyed a vanilla egg custard almost every day for the first three months after my surgery. If you are having a difficult time or are just nervous about eating solid foods for a while, try this custard.

My snacks of mozzarella string cheese were a lifesaver. Who would think that a little 1-ounce stick of cheese could be so satisfying? As long as we select lower-fat varieties, cheese is a great addition to our diets.

I began eating salads along with soft foods within three to four weeks of my surgery. Having a few tender leaves of baby lettuce with my tuna and shrimp purees satisfied my craving for vegetables. It is better to dress the entire bowl of greens rather than adding the dressing to individual servings. You use much less dressing, and you get better coverage when you toss the greens in a big bowl. This makes the greens very moist and easy to eat.

As you recuperate and progress, new foods may not always agree with you the first time you try them. If something doesn't go down well, try it again in a few days. I still make the shrimp, salmon, and tuna salads/purees in this section because they are delicious and provide an excellent protein lunch. I just leave them chunkier now and place a scoop on a bed of baby greens tossed with a little raspberry vinaigrette.

Remember that for the most part the serving counts given are for people who haven't had gastric bypass surgery. When a recipe serves 4, consider that a weight-loss surgery, or WLS, half portion is approximately half of a regular portion except where noted, and the nutritional counts are based on the smaller serving that is applicable to us.

stracciatella

WLS ½-cup portion: Calories 34, fat 2 gr, carbs <1 gr,
protein 3.5 gr
Makes 6 cups

Soothing first food when you return home from the hospital.
Make the homemade chicken stock base, and canned soup will
never taste the same again. So many people do not know how
to make chicken soup; if you are one of them, please give it a try
for this recipe. Make the stock before you have your surgery and
freeze it. When you are home, bring it to a boil and whisk in the
remaining ingredients.

6 cups homemade chicken stock (recipe follows)
3 large eggs
¼ cup freshly grated Parmesan
1 tablespoon finely chopped flat-leaf parsley
Pinch of freshly grated nutmeg
Kosher salt and freshly ground black pepper

Bring the stock to a boil in a large saucepan, then reduce the heat and
simmer. In a large bowl, beat the eggs with the Parmesan, parsley,
and nutmeg with a fork. Add the egg mixture to the broth in a steady
stream, stirring vigorously with the fork to break up the egg, which
will form fine, light flakes. Season with salt and pepper.

Note: If you need to use store-bought chicken or beef broth, Pacific, Imagine, or
Swanson Certified Organic are good brands that come in 1-quart "juice boxes"
(aseptic packaging). I also use Better Than Broth chicken, beef, mushroom,
lobster, or ham base (see Sources, page 303). One teaspoon of concentrated base
blends with 8 ounces of water to make a fast yet tasty stock.

chicken stock

*WLS ½-cup portion: Calories 40, fat 1.5 gr, carbs 4.0 gr,
protein 3.0 gr*
Makes about 4 quarts

After you have enjoyed the soup, use the chicken to make a basic
chicken salad, a perfect pureed protein food. Remove the tender
meat from the chicken once it has cooled and chop it very fine.
Don't use the food processor for your chicken salads; it will make
an unpalatable chicken paste. Moisten it with a little mayonnaise
and a tablespoon of your favorite bottled salad dressing (read
the label and make sure the dressing of your choice has less than
a gram or two of sugar and carbohydrates). You are looking for
a soft consistency as a recent post-op, so add a few spoonfuls of
chicken broth from the pot to further moisten the salad.

1 whole 2½- to 3-pound chicken
3 carrots, cut in half
3 celery stalks, cut in half
1 large onion, quartered
2 teaspoons kosher salt
½ teaspoon whole peppercorns

Place all the ingredients in an 8- to 10-quart stockpot and fill with
cold water to cover. Bring to a boil, then reduce the heat and simmer,
skimming any foam as necessary, for 3½ to 4 hours, until reduced by
about one third. Carefully transfer the chicken to a bowl and pour the
stock though a fine-mesh sieve set over a large bowl or pot, pressing
on the solids to extract as much liquid as possible. Cool the stock at
room temperature. Cover and chill until the fat has solidified, at least
overnight and up to 3 days. Scrape off and discard the fat.

cream of potato soup

WLS ½-cup portion: Calories 52, fat <1 gr, carbs 9.5 gr, protein 3.5 gr
Makes 6 cups

An excellent first post-op food. An immersion blender allows you to make a smooth soup or sauce right in the pot. If you are within days of your surgery, you will be consuming about ½ cup of soup, so note that the carbohydrate count is calculated accordingly.

3½ cups diced Yukon gold potatoes, peeled, about 1½ pounds or 4 medium potatoes
½ small onion, chopped
1 medium shallot, sliced
1 quart Chicken Stock (page 128) or chicken broth
¼ teaspoon dried thyme
Kosher salt and freshly ground black pepper
½ cup 1% low-fat milk
Shredded Cheddar, for serving

Combine the potatoes, onion, shallot, stock, thyme, ½ teaspoon salt, and a few grinds of black pepper in a medium saucepan. Bring to a boil, reduce the heat, and simmer for 15 to 20 minutes, until the potatoes are fork tender. Puree the potato-stock mixture with an immersion blender or in a blender until smooth and creamy. Be careful when pureeing hot liquids in a blender as the steam expands; always cover the lid with a kitchen towel, pulse the switch, then release the steam before proceeding.

Reheat just before serving; add the milk and season with salt and pepper. Top each serving with 1 tablespoon of shredded Cheddar.

creamy black bean soup

WLS ½-cup portion: Calories 62, fat 2.5 gr, carbs 7.5 gr, protein 3.5 gr
Makes 6 cups

This smooth hot soup will be comforting to both you and your family. A tossed salad and a plate of Cheddar quesadillas with pickled jalapeños round out the meal. This thin but flavorful soup was created for use early after surgery; later on you can add a second can of black beans for a heartier version.

1 tablespoon olive oil
1 small onion, chopped
2 garlic cloves, chopped
One 15-ounce can black beans, rinsed and drained
3 cups Chicken Stock (page 128) or low-sodium chicken broth
½ cup mild roasted-tomato salsa (see Note)
Kosher salt and freshly ground black pepper
½ cup reduced-fat sour cream
Shredded Cheddar, chopped cilantro, and sliced green onions
**   (scallions), for serving**

Heat the oil in a large, heavy saucepan over medium heat. Sauté the onion and garlic until lightly browned, about 4 minutes. Add the beans, stock, and salsa, and season with salt and pepper. Bring the soup to a boil, reduce the heat, and simmer for 10 minutes, stirring occasionally, until the flavors blend and the soup thickens slightly. Puree the soup with an immersion blender or in a blender until smooth and creamy. Be careful when pureeing hot liquids in a blender as the steam expands; always cover the lid with a kitchen towel, pulse the switch, then release the steam before proceeding.

Reheat the soup just before serving and whisk in the sour cream. Check the seasonings. Ladle the soup into bowls and garnish with the Cheddar, cilantro, and green onions. Have a bottle of hot sauce on the table and use to taste.

Note: Rick Bayless, chef/owner of Chicago's Topolobampo and Frontera Grill, is the hand behind the Frontera and Salpica brands of salsa—they are absolutely delicious. Newman's Own and Goya salsas are also excellent. Watch for added sugar in other brands.

italian tomato soup

WLS ½-cup portion: Calories 54, fat 1 gr, carbs 5 gr, protein 4 gr
Makes 4 cups

A simple, smooth, and satisfying soup that you can put together in minutes. Excellent for your early pureed food stage, but delicious enough that it will be a family favorite. Serve with a grilled cheese sandwich and it is a fast after-work meal for your family.

One 29-ounce can whole tomatoes with juice
One 15-ounce can navy or cannellini beans, rinsed and drained
1 teaspoon dried basil
2 tablespoons grated Parmesan
½ teaspoon garlic powder
Kosher salt and freshly ground black pepper

Place the tomatoes, beans, basil, Parmesan cheese, and garlic powder in a blender and puree until very smooth. Pour into a medium saucepan, bring to a boil, reduce the heat, and simmer for 20 minutes, stirring occasionally. Season with salt and pepper.

creamy tuscan bean soup

WLS ½-cup portion: Calories 105, fat 3 gr, carbs 8 gr, protein 5 gr
Makes 4 cups

When my aunt Gail and I traveled through Tuscany we had many versions of traditional bean soup during the primo, or first, course. The creaminess and ease of preparation make this a staple of the pureed and then the soft diet, but it is so good that you will make it as a quick supper on many occasions. Serve with a tossed salad and sliced Italian bread.

Two 15-ounce cans great northern or cannelini beans, drained
1½ cups Chicken Stock (page 128) or canned broth
   (see Note, page 127)
2 garlic cloves, whole
¼ teaspoon dried rosemary
¼ teaspoon dried thyme
⅛ teaspoon crushed red pepper flakes
2 tablespoons extra-virgin olive oil
Kosher salt and freshly ground black pepper

Place the beans, stock, garlic, rosemary, thyme, and red pepper flakes in a blender. Puree until smooth. Pour into a medium saucepan, add the olive oil, bring to a boil, lower the heat, and simmer for 20 minutes. Season with salt and pepper. Ladle into bowls.

french onion soup

WLS ½-cup portion: Calories 65.5, fat 2.5 gr, carbs 5 gr,
protein 2.5 gr
Makes 6 cups

Another basic soup to have in your repertoire while relearning
to eat after surgery. It is very simple to make and enjoyable to
sip. Turkey sandwiches on hard rolls with lettuce and tomato
complete a family meal. If you are less than two months post-op,
you may wish to omit the cheese from your portion, as it may be
too difficult to chew into a smooth mouthful.

1 tablespoon salted butter
1 tablespoon olive oil
2 medium white onions, chopped, about 1½ pounds
2 medium red onions, chopped, about 1½ pounds
2 garlic cloves, chopped
1 cup white wine
1 quart beef broth (see Note, page 127)
2 cups chicken broth (see Note, page 127)
½ teaspoon Tabasco sauce
1 teaspoon Worcestershire sauce
¼ teaspoon freshly grated nutmeg
Kosher salt and freshly ground black pepper
½ cup finely shredded Swiss cheese, about ⅛ pound

Heat the butter and olive oil in a large, heavy pot over medium-low
heat. Sauté the onions and garlic until very soft and brown, about
30 minutes, stirring frequently. Add the wine and continue to cook
until the mixture is reduced to a thick glaze. Stir in the beef broth,

before

chicken broth, Tabasco, Worcestershire, and nutmeg. Reduce the heat and simmer for 45 minutes. Season with salt and pepper.

To serve, reheat the soup to boiling, ladle into bowls, and sprinkle with some of the cheese.

hummus

WLS ¼-cup portion: Calories 65.5, fat 4 gr, carbs 6.4 gr, protein 2 gr
Makes 2 cups

Eating right after surgery can be a chore. It is hard to find foods that are smooth and palatable and have some protein value. I loved homemade hummus before my surgery, so it was a natural to give it a try post-op. It is smooth and flavorful and later on is an excellent side dish for a grilled shrimp or chicken skewer.

One 16-ounce can chickpeas, rinsed and drained
3 garlic cloves, thinly sliced
⅓ cup tahini (sesame paste)
2 tablespoons fresh lemon juice (about 1 lemon)
2 tablespoons extra-virgin olive oil
Kosher salt and freshly ground black pepper
2 tablespoons coarsely chopped flat-leaf parsley

In a food processor or blender, puree the chickpeas with the garlic, tahini, lemon juice, olive oil, and as much water as necessary to process the hummus to a smooth mayonnaise-like consistency, scraping down the sides to incorporate all the chickpeas. Add salt and pepper to taste and transfer to a bowl. Sprinkle with the parsley.

pinto bean dip

WLS ¼-cup portion: Calories 59, fat 2 gr, carbs 8 gr, protein 2.5 gr
Makes 2 cups

Another smooth, easy-to-digest puree. Make turkey burgers or hamburgers on soft sesame-seed rolls for the rest of the family, serving this dish as a "refried bean" side dish with a dollop of sour cream, extra cheese, and a few pickled jalapeño slices.

1 small onion, minced
2 garlic cloves, minced
1 tablespoon olive oil
One 16-ounce can pinto beans, rinsed and drained
½ to 1 cup Chicken Stock canned or broth (see Note, page 127)
¼ teaspoon ground cumin
Kosher salt and freshly ground black pepper
1 tablespoon finely chopped cilantro
½ cup shredded Cheddar, about ¼ pound

Sauté the onion and garlic in the oil in a large nonstick skillet over medium-high heat, stirring constantly until lightly browned and very soft, about 6 minutes. Add the beans and mash with a potato masher or the back of a large wooden spoon to make a coarse puree. Stir in enough broth to thin to a creamy consistency. Continue to cook, stirring occasionally, until the mixture is hot. Add the cumin and season with salt and pepper. Remove from the heat and stir in the cilantro and Cheddar.

shrimp salad spread

WLS ½-cup portion: Calories 115, fat 7 gr, carbs <1 gr,
protein 12 gr
Makes 2½ cups

I practically live on this shrimp salad, even eleven years after
my bariatric surgery. It is extremely moist, high in protein, and
extraordinarily delicious. I sauté a pound of shrimp, mix it up
with the remaining ingredients in my mini food processor, and
keep it in a bowl in my refrigerator for quick lunches and suppers,
or even for a snack if I am so inclined. I don't snack often, but
I know that a couple of tablespoons of shrimp salad on a melba
round is better than a handful of Fritos or crackers, which will
destroy my carbohydrate count for the day.

Early after my surgery I pureed this into a smooth shrimp
paste, but now I leave it much chunkier and use more Old Bay
seasoning to spice it up. I toss a handful of mixed baby greens
with a little dressing and put my portion of shrimp salad on top.
Sautéing the shrimp in a bit of olive oil rather than poaching or
boiling them in water concentrates the flavor of the seafood and
gives it another layer of taste.

½ teaspoon olive oil
1 pound medium shrimp, peeled and deveined
¼ cup light mayonnaise (see Note)
Juice of ½ lemon, about 1 tablespoon
2 green onions (scallions), sliced, including the green tops
1 teaspoon Old Bay Seasoning

Heat the olive oil in a large nonstick skillet over medium-high heat.
Add the shrimp and sauté for 2 to 3 minutes, stirring constantly,

until just opaque throughout. Transfer to a small bowl and set aside. Blend the mayonnaise, lemon juice, green onions, and Old Bay Seasoning in a food processor until smooth; add the shrimp and pulse until they are very finely chopped and the mixture is well blended. Transfer to a serving bowl, cover, and chill.

Note: I prefer Hellmann's mayonnaise. They make regular, light, and reduced-fat versions.

mediterranean tuna spread

WLS ½-cup portion: Calories 85, fat 3.5 gr, carbs <1 gr,
protein 11 gr
Makes 2½ cups

Tuna is another mainstay of my diet! The new pouches of tuna have a fresh taste and are so much more flavorful than the canned variety; give them a try. Since they are packed without the addition of water, I add a little chicken broth or water for a moister consistency.

Two 6-ounce pouches albacore tuna
2 tablespoons reduced-fat mayonnaise
Juice of 1 lemon, about 2 tablespoons
2 tablespoons drained and finely chopped roasted red peppers
10 Kalamata or oil-cured olives, pitted and finely chopped (see Note)
2 tablespoons finely minced red onion
Kosher salt and freshly ground black pepper

Empty the tuna into a small bowl and mash with a fork until very finely flaked. Add the mayonnaise, lemon juice, roasted peppers, olives, and onion and stir to combine, adding a little water or chicken broth to further moisten. Add salt and pepper to taste.

Note: It is becoming more common to find displays of olives in many markets, and any black olive that appeals to you will work in this recipe. Smash the olives with the flat side of a large knife. The pit will easily come away from the olive.

curried chicken and almond spread

WLS ½-cup portion: Calories 113, fat 7 gr, carbs 1 gr, protein 11 gr
Makes 2½ cups

I make this salad with the chicken left over from a pot of chicken stock. Transfer the whole chicken to a large bowl, allow it to cool, and remove and discard the bones and the skin. Finely chop the chicken meat with a knife. A food processor will turn the tender meat into a blob of unpalatable chicken paste. This is also a great salad to make with a take-out rotisserie chicken. Serve a small scoop of dressed baby greens on top.

1½ teaspoons curry powder
2 tablespoons light mayonnaise
2 tablespoons nonfat yogurt
Juice of 1 lemon, about 2 tablespoons
Kosher salt and freshly ground black pepper
2 cups very finely chopped cooked chicken
1 tablespoon minced red onion
1 tablespoon minced flat-leaf parsley

1 tablespoon finely chopped almonds
2 to 3 tablespoons chicken broth (see Note, page 127)

Toast the curry powder in a small skillet over medium heat until a wisp of smoke appears and the mixture is fragrant, about 30 seconds. Transfer to a medium bowl and blend with the mayonnaise, yogurt, and lemon juice, and season with salt and pepper. Add the chicken, onion, parsley, and almonds; blend until the mixture is well combined, adding a little broth to moisten further.

salmon salad

WLS ½-cup portion: Calories 91, fat 3.5 gr, carbs 2.5 gr, protein 12.5 gr
Makes 2½ cups

Salmon is high in protein, readily available, and moist and tender to eat. Roast a double portion of salmon for dinner and chill the leftovers to make this salad for the next day's lunch.

1 pound cooked salmon fillet, skin and bones removed, then chilled
3 green onions (scallions), minced
¼ cup bottled raspberry-balsamic dressing (see Note), or Sesame Dressing (page 219)
Kosher salt and freshly ground black pepper
Baby spinach, rinsed and dried

Flake the salmon into fine pieces. Add the green onions and salad dressing and gently combine with the salmon mixture. Add salt and pepper to taste. Serve a small portion on top of a bed of lightly dressed baby spinach leaves.

Note: Consorzio is a flavorful brand of raspberry-balsamic dressing that I use regularly (see Sources, page 303).

turkey tomato ragù

WLS ½-cup portion: Calories 107, fat 5.5 gr, carbs 4 gr, protein 11 gr
Serves 4 when used as pasta sauce

This thick, meaty, chili-type dish is very easy to eat when you first try different pureed and soft foods. If you mash the turkey with a fork while it is browning, you will end up with a very fine-textured mixture to eat by the spoonful. Cook some ziti or bow-tie pasta and use the remaining ragù as a sauce for the rest of the family.

1 teaspoon olive oil
1 pound ground turkey breast (see Note)
1 garlic clove, minced
1 small red onion, minced
One 14-ounce can tomato sauce
2 teaspoons dried basil
½ teaspoon dried oregano
½ teaspoon dried thyme
Kosher salt and freshly ground black pepper

Heat the olive oil in a deep skillet over medium-high heat. Brown the turkey, mashing with a wooden spoon or fork to break up chunks. Add the garlic and onion and cook until softened, stirring occasionally. Stir in the tomato sauce and 1 cup water, then add the basil, oregano, and thyme, and season with salt and pepper. Cover and simmer over low heat for 20 minutes, or until the flavors are blended.

Note: I have substituted a high-protein soy crumble product for the turkey and it is nearly indistinguishable.

Variation: This recipe can also go Mexican with the substitution of 2 teaspoons of chili powder for the basil. Serve it in a deep bowl ladled over a scoop of white rice and sprinkled with sliced green onions.

double chocolate super protein pudding

WLS ½-cup portion: Calories 60, fat 0 gr, carbs 3 gr, protein 10 gr
Makes 4 (½-cup) servings

This is one of my favorite discoveries for the new and greatly improved ready-to-drink protein shakes on the market. Use one of our smooth and creamy RTDs in place of milk and turn an ordinary package of Jell-O Sugar-Free Instant Pudding mix into a super protein-packed pudding that is absolutely delicious. Mix and match flavors: lemon or pistachio pudding mix with Vanilla Micellar Milk, banana pudding mix with Banana Worldwide Pure Protein Shake, butterscotch pudding mix with Praline Scream Extreme Smoothie; get creative.

2 cups Micellar Milk ready-to-drink protein shake
One package (1 ounce) Jell-O Sugar-free Instant Pudding Mix, chocolate

Beat pudding mix into the cold ready-to-drink protein in a deep bowl with a wire whisk for 2 minutes. Pour at once into individual serving dishes. Pudding will be soft-set and ready to eat within 5 minutes.

cinnamon applesauce

WLS ¼-cup portion: Calories 31, fat 0 gr, carbs 6.5 gr,
protein <1 gr
Makes about 4 cups

Homemade cinnamon applesauce is an ideal texture for even
early post-ops; smells like heaven, and is super-easy for even a
noncook. Make a big batch; your family will eat it up. Blend your
delicious applesauce with unflavored yogurt, cottage or ricotta
cheese, or use to sauce thinly sliced roasted turkey tenderloin or
chicken thighs.

8 large apples *(I use a blend of apples as they cook down with*
   different textures; McIntosh for smooth sauce, Fuji for chunky,
   Granny Smith for tart)
½ teaspoon cinnamon
½ cup Splenda granular, plus additional to taste

Cut each apple into quarters; peel skin and remove core of each piece.
Place prepared apples into a large covered saucepan, add cinnamon,
and ¼ cup of water. Cover pan, bring to a boil, lower heat to a simmer and cook apples 30 to 40 minutes, until very soft. Remove from
heat, and mash apples into a chunky sauce using a potato masher or a
wooden spoon. If you are a very early post-op, use a blender or food
processor to turn apples into a smooth puree. Stir in ½ cup Splenda,
plus additional if needed, to taste. Serve warm or chilled.

vanilla egg custard

WLS ½-cup portion: Calories 110, fat 4.5 gr, carbs 7.5 gr, protein 9 gr
Makes six ½-cup servings

This custard is smooth, cold, and very soothing. I made a batch at least twice a week, as my family loved this as well. Purchase six or eight 4-ounce custard cups; they are invaluable for portion control.

4 large eggs
1 cup skim milk
1½ cups evaporated low-fat milk
½ cup Splenda Granular
2 teaspoons vanilla extract
Pinch of kosher salt
Freshly grated nutmeg

Preheat the oven to 325°F. Place 6 custard cups or ramekins in a large roasting pan and set aside. Whisk together the eggs, milk, evaporated milk, Splenda, vanilla, and salt. Pour through a fine-mesh sieve into a large measuring cup. Divide evenly among the custard cups and grate a generous amount of nutmeg over each one. Pour enough hot water in the roasting pan to come about halfway up the sides of the custard cups. Bake for 25 to 35 minutes, until the custards are just set in the center. Carefully remove the custards from the water bath, and transfer to a wire rack to cool. Serve chilled.

green chile cheese puff
with roasted tomato salsa

WLS ½ portion: Calories 163, fat 10 gr, carbs 6 gr, protein 12 gr
Serves 4

This dinner is full of protein and flavor, while the salsa accompaniment makes the soufflé extra moist. While the soufflé-like puff bakes, I make a salad of mixed baby greens, sliced grape tomatoes, thin cucumber slices, and red onions, and toss it with store-bought ranch dressing. A handful of golden baked pita chips or homemade baked flatbread wedges rounds out the meal for the family.

roasted-tomato salsa

4 large ripe Roma tomatoes, cut in half lengthwise
1 garlic clove, peeled and left whole
1 small red onion, peeled and sliced
1 jalapeño chile, cut in half lengthwise, stemmed, and seeded
Juice of 1 lime, about 1½ tablespoons
1 tablespoon olive oil
2 tablespoons chopped cilantro
Kosher salt and freshly ground black pepper

green chile cheese puff

Vegetable oil cooking spray
¼ cup all-purpose flour
¾ teaspoon kosher salt
½ teaspoon baking powder
6 large eggs

2 tablespoons salted butter, melted
1 cup 2% low-fat cottage cheese
1 cup freshly shredded medium-sharp Cheddar, about ¼ pound
Two 4-ounce cans diced mild green chiles, drained

Preheat the broiler to the highest temperature. Line a baking sheet with foil, folding up the edges to catch the juices. Arrange the tomatoes, garlic, onion slices, and jalapeño on the baking sheet and broil for 8 minutes, or until the vegetables are lightly charred and softened. Lift the foil, being careful to keep the juices, and pour into a blender or food processor. Add the lime juice, olive oil, and cilantro, and pulse the mixture until it is an even consistency but not completely smooth. Season with salt and pepper and set aside.

Preheat the oven to 350°F. Lightly coat a 9-inch glass pie plate with cooking spray. Sift together the flour, salt, and baking powder into a small bowl and set aside. Beat the eggs in a large bowl with an electric mixer until doubled in volume, about 4 minutes. Blend in the flour mixture and melted butter. Stir in the cottage cheese, Cheddar, and green chiles. Pour the mixture into the prepared pie plate. Bake the custard in the middle of the oven for 30 to 40 minutes, until the top is puffed and golden brown and a sharp knife inserted near the center comes out clean. Cut the cheese puff into wedges and spoon some of the roasted-tomato salsa over each piece.

sunday morning frittata

WLS ½ portion: Calories 130, fat 8 gr, carbs 4 gr, protein 11 gr
Serves 4

Packed with protein and soft enough to eat very early in your post-op period. Be creative with your choice of vegetables and

cheese, keeping track of the carbohydrate count. Serve for
breakfast with fresh melon or a berry compote, or for supper with
a tossed salad.

1 tablespoon salted butter
1 small zucchini, finely diced
8 mushrooms, finely diced
6 large eggs
½ cup 1% low-fat milk
1 cup 2% low-fat cottage cheese
1 cup shredded Jarlsberg or Swiss cheese, about ¼ pound
3 green onions (scallions), sliced
1 ripe Roma tomato, diced
1 tablespoon chopped fresh dill
Vegetable oil cooking spray

Preheat the oven to 350°F. Heat the butter in a medium nonstick skillet and lightly sauté the zucchini and mushrooms until the released
juices have reduced and the vegetables are lightly browned. In a large
bowl, beat the eggs with the milk until well blended, then stir in the
cottage cheese, Jarlsberg cheese, green onions, tomato, dill, and the
sautéed vegetables. Pour into a 9 × 9-inch baking dish that has been
lightly coated with cooking spray. Bake for 40 to 45 minutes, until a
knife inserted near the center comes out clean.

If using 4 individual ramekins, place them on a baking sheet and
bake for 25 to 30 minutes, until still a bit soft in the center.

mexican meatball soup

WLS ½-cup portion: Calories 79, fat 4 gr, carbs 5.5 gr,
protein 5.5 gr
Makes six 1-cup servings

This soup works at all post-op food stages. In the early stages, eat
a couple of the tiny meatballs for a little protein. I serve my family
some quesadilla wedges made with pepper Jack cheese and a
bowl of homemade guacamole.

1 tablespoon olive oil
1 large sweet onion, finely diced
4 garlic cloves, minced
1 bay leaf
1 quart Chicken Stock or canned broth (see Note, page 127)
One 16-ounce can diced tomatoes (see Note)
½ cup medium-hot tomato salsa (see Note, page 131)
¾ cup chopped cilantro
½ pound ground turkey breast
2 tablespoons minced red onion
2 tablespoons yellow cornmeal
3 tablespoons skim milk
1 large egg
¼ teaspoon ground cumin
Kosher salt and freshly ground black pepper
Tabasco sauce

Heat the oil in large pot over medium-high heat. Add the onion, half
of the garlic, and the bay leaf and sauté until very soft and golden
brown, about 8 minutes. Add the stock, tomatoes with juice, salsa,

and about one third of the cilantro. Bring to a boil, then cover, reduce the heat, and simmer for 15 minutes.

Combine the turkey, red onion, cornmeal, milk, egg, cumin, ½ teaspoon salt, a few grinds of black pepper, the remaining garlic, and another third of the cilantro, blending well. Shape the meat by rolling generous tablespoons into 1-inch balls. Add the meatballs to the soup and bring to a low boil, stirring occasionally. Cover the soup, reduce the heat, and simmer for 20 minutes. Season with salt, pepper, and Tabasco; stir in the remaining cilantro. Discard the bay leaf before serving.

Note: If you can find Muir Glen Fire Roasted Tomatoes, use them in this soup. They are also excellent for many other recipes in this book.

light manicotti

WLS portion of ½ manicotti: Calories 96, fat 4.5 gr, carbs 6.6 gr, protein 7 gr
Makes 10 pieces of manicotti

Italian comfort food that is also very soft and easy to eat. I don't eat pasta anymore; it has too many carbohydrates and gives me an uncomfortably full feeling even in small amounts, but I do enjoy these tender, cheese-filled egg crepes. I make this dish for Sunday dinner and everyone is happy. You can use the Italian Meatballs recipe on page 235 to add to the sauce for this recipe. Serve your manicotti with a tossed salad dressed with balsamic vinegar and olive oil along with a loaf of Italian bread.

sauce

1 tablespoon olive oil
1 small onion, diced
2 garlic cloves, minced
One 28-ounce can crushed Italian tomatoes
One 4-ounce can tomato paste
1 tablespoon dried basil
½ teaspoon dried oregano
½ teaspoon dried thyme
¼ teaspoon crushed red pepper flakes
Kosher salt and freshly ground black pepper

crepes

1 cup all-purpose flour
½ cup 1% low-fat milk
3 large eggs
½ teaspoon kosher salt
Olive oil or vegetable oil cooking spray

filling

1 pound part-skim ricotta
½ cup shredded part-skim mozzarella, plus additional for topping
¼ cup freshly grated Parmesan
2 large eggs
3 tablespoons chopped flat-leaf parsley

Heat the olive oil in a large saucepan over medium-high heat. Sauté the onion and garlic until softened. Add the tomatoes, tomato paste, and 1 cup water. Stir in the basil, oregano, thyme, and red pepper flakes, season with salt and pepper, bring the sauce to a boil, then reduce the heat and simmer while preparing the crepes and filling.

In a large bowl, blend the flour, milk, eggs, and salt until smooth. Heat an 8-inch nonstick skillet over medium heat and lightly grease with a few drops of olive oil or cooking spray. Ladle 2 tablespoons of the batter into the center of the pan. Lift the pan from the burner and swirl it so the batter smoothly coats the entire bottom. Replace the pan on the burner and cook just until the surface looks dry. Using a spatula or your fingers, flip the crepe and cook for a few seconds until the other side is lightly browned. Repeat with the remaining batter to make 10 crepes.

Preheat the oven to 375°F. Blend the ricotta, mozzarella, and Parmesan with the eggs and parsley. Spoon the filling into a large plastic bag, squeeze out the air, and snip about ½ inch off of one corner. Spread 1 cup of the tomato sauce on the bottom of a large shallow baking dish. Lay a crepe on a flat surface, pipe about ¼ cup of the filling in a thick line down the center by squeezing the bag, then roll the crepe, tucking in the sides. Place the rolled crepe in the prepared baking dish, seam side down. Repeat with the remaining crepes. Cover the crepes with tomato sauce, sprinkle with mozzarella, and bake for 40 minutes, or until hot and bubbling.

cottage cheese pancakes

Per 2 pancakes: Calories 98, fat 6 gr, carbs 4 gr, protein 8 gr
Makes 8 pancakes

These are delicious: warm and cheesy, with bits of fried onion!
Surprisingly good, given that the recipe contains just five

ingredients. Double or triple this recipe to make enough for
the family, as everyone will love these! Bake rounds of pancetta
(Italian cured bacon) on a baking sheet for 10 minutes, or until
crisp, to serve with the pancakes for a tasty brunch.

½ medium onion, chopped
2 tablespoons butter
Kosher salt and freshly ground black pepper
2 eggs
1 cup cottage cheese
3 tablespoons all-purpose flour
Vegetable oil cooking spray

Sauté the onion in the butter until golden and season with salt and
pepper. In a small bowl, combine the eggs, cottage cheese, flour, salt
and pepper, and the cooked onion mixture. Spray a nonstick skillet
with vegetable oil cooking spray. For each pancake, scoop 2 tablespoons of batter into the skillet and coax into a 3-inch round. Cook
until the undersides are golden brown, 2 to 3 minutes. Flip and cook
for 1 to 2 minutes longer or until lightly browned. Transfer to a baking sheet and keep warm in a 200°F oven.

supreme pizza bake

WLS ½-cup serving: Calories 169, fat 9.3 gr, carbs 4 gr,
protein 17 gr
Serves 8

This is my answer to the many requests for a post-op pizza.
I have taken the ingredients of pizza and combined them with
a lasagna-like ricotta cheese layer to add protein and lighten

up the meat. Use any combination of pizza toppings that your family likes, but I do love the sausage and pepperoni. The addition of whole fennel seed really adds amazing flavor, so please don't think it isn't essential. Serve this cheesy bake with a big green salad. Anyone who loves pizza will love this dish.

While this is a soft food in texture, it does contain ground and chopped meats, which makes it a more advanced soft food recipe and not a first food.

2 cups marinara sauce (I prefer Gia Russa Hot Sicilian sauce)
8 ounces lean Italian sausage (Jimmy Dean is a very lean brand)
¼ teaspoon whole fennel seed
½ cup diced pepperoni slices
15 ounces part-skim ricotta
1 large egg
¼ cup grated Parmesan
½ cup roasted red peppers
2 cups shredded mozzarella
¼ teaspoon crushed red pepper flakes
½ teaspoon dried oregano

Preheat the oven to 350°F.

Pour half of the sauce into a 2-quart casserole dish. Brown the sausage in a nonstick skillet, mashing with a fork while cooking for a fine texture; blend in the fennel seed. Add the pepperoni and cook until the fat is rendered, 2 to 4 minutes. Transfer the meat mixture to the casserole dish using a slotted spoon to drain the fat. Blend the ricotta with the egg and half of the Parmesan cheese in a small bowl and spread evenly over the meat layer. Arrange the roasted peppers on top and spoon on the remaining marinara sauce. Evenly spread the shredded mozzarella and sprinkle with the remaining Parmesan cheese and the red pepper flakes and oregano.

Bake for 35 to 40 minutes, until bubbling and hot in the center.
Allow the casserole to cool for 10 minutes before serving.

bacon and swiss cheese pie

*WLS "crustless" serving: Calories 214, fat 11 gr, carbs 4 gr,
protein 19 gr*
Serves 6

It is good to know how to bake a basic quiche! When we have
family for a holiday or weekend it is difficult to cook a big
breakfast for the crowd. However, I can quickly assemble two
of these pies and while they bake I have plenty of time to set
the table and cut up melon and berries for fresh fruit salad.
This delicious pie also works well for a supper, and leftovers
are a perfect lunch when reheated in the office microwave. I
just eat the delicious cheese and bacon custard and leave the
crust.

The nutmeg adds an unbelievable spark of traditional flavor,
so don't leave it out.

**One 9-inch unbaked pie crust, homemade or store-bought frozen
prepared (I use Mrs. Smiths)**
4 slices bacon
2 cups shredded Swiss cheese
5 large eggs
1 cup whole milk
½ teaspoon kosher salt
¼ teaspoon freshly ground black pepper
¼ teaspoon freshly ground nutmeg

Place the pan containing the pie crust on a baking sheet and preheat the oven to 350°F.

Cut the bacon crosswise into ¼-inch-thick pieces. Cook the bacon in a nonstick skillet over medium heat until golden and crisp. Drain on a paper towel and reserve. Spread the Swiss cheese evenly on the bottom of the pie crust, and then sprinkle with the bacon pieces.

Whisk together the eggs and milk until thoroughly blended. Stir in the salt, pepper, and nutmeg. Pour over the bacon and cheese in the crust.

Bake for 35 to 40 minutes, until the filling is golden and puffed and cooked throughout. The pie is done if there are no waves moving across the center of the pie when jiggled, or if a sharp knife blade is clean when inserted near the center of the pie. Serve warm.

eggs poached in
spicy tomato sauce

Per 1-egg serving: Calories 157, fat 12 gr, carbs 3.5 gr,
protein 10 gr
Makes 4 eggs

Eggs are a quick-cooking and excellent source of protein that are tender and easy to eat when simmered in a sauce or when cooked in an omelet. It is common for scrambled eggs not to be easily tolerated for post-ops due to the pebbly texture. The technique demonstrated in this recipe is a kitchen classic, and I will often poach eggs for myself using a jar of fire-roasted salsa or a bottle of Gia Russa–brand spaghetti sauce when I get home from work and need to prepare dinner quickly with an almost bare pantry.

2 slices bacon, cut crosswise into ½-inch pieces

2 garlic cloves, chopped

1 tablespoon chopped chipotle chiles in adobo sauce (in a can in
   the Latin section)

One 28-ounce can chef's cut or diced tomatoes in puree or juice,
   undrained

Kosher salt and freshly ground black pepper

4 large eggs

¼ cup crumbled feta cheese

Sauté the bacon in a nonstick skillet until golden and crisp, about
4 minutes; transfer to a paper towel and set aside. Add the garlic
and chiles to the rendered fat in the skillet and cook until the garlic
is golden. Add the tomatoes and juice and simmer the mixture over
medium heat until thickened, 15 to 20 minutes. Season with salt and
pepper.

Reduce the heat to low. Break a single egg into a small cup. Make
a slight hole in the sauce with the back of a large spoon and slip the
egg into the hole. Repeat with the remaining eggs. Cover and cook
very gently for 6 to 9 minutes, until the egg whites are opaque but
the yolks are soft. Spoon into bowls with sauce and sprinkle with feta
and bacon.

fish and seafood

Most post-op weight-loss surgery people will tell you that seafood is the perfect food for them to eat because of the soft, moist texture, high protein, and low fat content. Fish contains about 7 grams of protein per ounce, so a 5-ounce serving of broiled grouper has 35 grams of protein! Top that with charred tomato vinaigrette to further moisten the fish and you have a dinner that's suitable even for guests.

I have always loved seafood, so it has been easy for me to leave the sirloin behind and concentrate on shrimp and swordfish. If you can't find the particular fish suggested in the recipe, substitute one with a similar texture. A large percentage of WLS people have never cooked seafood because its purchase and preparation intimidate many novice cooks. If you follow a few basic guidelines, you will be able to prepare many of these recipes in less than 30 minutes.

Smell is the key indicator of freshness. Fresh fish has a clean, bright, fresh smell. Don't buy it if it has a "fishy" or ammonia odor. I usually buy my fish in a specialty fish market where I have a better guarantee of quality. Once the folks behind the counter get to know you, they will recommend what just came in, or guide you to which catch is of exceptional quality. If you do not live in an area where fresh fish is readily available, check your frozen food section for individually frozen salmon and tilapia fillets, peeled and cleaned raw shrimp, and scallops. They will be perfectly fresh and work well in these recipes.

The secret to moist fish is to not overcook it. The general rule of thumb is to cook fish 8 to 10 minutes per inch of thickness, measuring the fillet or steak at its thickest point. So, a salmon fillet approximately one inch thick should be cooked for no more than 8 to 10 minutes total. Sauté a much thinner ¼-inch flounder fillet for only 2 to 3 minutes. I keep a ruler in my kitchen gadget drawer to help estimate cooking times.

We can also rely on seafood when eating in restaurants. I no longer hesitate when faced with an impromptu lunch or dinner situation. I know I can find a protein source that works for me, such as a salmon Caesar salad, tuna melt, or shrimp cocktail, on any menu. When ordering from a menu you have to think about what the texture will be when you chew a bite of the food; a bite of grilled salmon with mango salsa will always be moister than a bite of roasted chicken breast.

Several of my first restaurant meals when I was six to eight weeks post-op were at our favorite sushi bar. I was a bit nervous, but with a little thought I was able to put together a perfect sushi dinner. I picked apart some of the rolls, ate only the fish from my sushi, and had a very successful first outing. Since my sushi chef noticed that I was leaving the rice and the seaweed wrappers, he has created a roll for me that is perfect for WLS sushi lovers. The nori wrappers were too tough for me to chew really well at first, so he made a small roll using a sheet of moistened rice paper, with chopped spicy tuna, avocado slices, scallions, and a spicy Japanese mayonnaise dipping sauce. He also prepared raw tuna and yellowtail for me sashimi-style in paper-thin slices that I dip in ponzu sauce. Everything is very tender and easy to chew and tastes great. I do not eat rice, since it is too high in carbohydrates and would fill me up before I got to my protein.

These seafood recipes serve four people who have not had gastric bypass surgery. The person who is eating after having had bypass surgery would be eating about half of one serving. For example, a recipe using 1½ pounds of shrimp would feed 4 people with a 6-ounce portion per person; the WLS half portion would be a 3-ounce portion with enough of the sauce to moisten it. The nutritional analysis has been calculated for the WLS half portion including the sauce or salsa for that dish.

mykonos shrimp with feta

WLS ½ portion: Calories 207, fat 10 gr, carbs 8 gr, protein 18 gr
Serves 4

Shrimp are incredibly moist, making them texturally one of the easiest proteins to eat after surgery. They are my favorite food! I keep bags of raw, flash-frozen, peeled, and deveined shrimp in the freezer, so this is a quick meal to prepare when I'm running late. I thaw the frozen shrimp in a bowl of cool water and by the time the remaining ingredients are prepared, the shrimp will be defrosted.

When I make this dish for a special occasion, I use individual, hand-painted baking dishes that can go under the broiler so each guest gets his or her own portion. A salad of baby spinach leaves tossed with oil-cured olives and red onions, dressed with a little lemon juice and olive oil, completes this meal.

1 large onion, thinly sliced
3 garlic cloves, thinly sliced
3 tablespoons olive oil
One 14-ounce can diced tomatoes, drained (see Note, page 148)
½ cup white wine
1 teaspoon dried oregano
⅛ teaspoon ground cinnamon

Kosher salt and freshly ground black pepper

½ cup chopped flat-leaf parsley

1½ pounds large shrimp, peeled and deveined

2 medium tomatoes, peeled with a vegetable peeler then
    thinly sliced

¼ pound Greek feta cheese, rinsed, drained, and crumbled

Preheat the oven to 450°F. Sauté the onion and garlic in 1 table-spoon of the olive oil in a nonstick skillet over medium-high heat until golden brown. Add the tomatoes, wine, oregano, and cinnamon; lightly season with salt and pepper and cook until most of the liquid has evaporated, about 12 minutes. Stir in half of the parsley and spoon the sauce evenly over the bottom of a decorative baking dish. Sauté the shrimp in another tablespoon of the olive oil in a nonstick skillet over high heat until they just begin to turn pink and curl, about 2 minutes. Arrange the shrimp on top of the sauce in the baking dish, add a layer of the sliced tomatoes and then the feta; drizzle with the remaining tablespoon of olive oil and a few grinds of black pepper. Bake for 15 to 18 minutes, until the sauce is bubbling. Turn the broiler to high and cook for an additional 1 to 2 minutes, until the feta is golden. Garnish with the remaining parsley and serve immediately.

bengal shrimp korma

WLS ½ portion: Calories 103, fat 3 gr, carbs 3 gr, protein 15 gr
Serves 4

This Indian combination can be thrown together in minutes
if you have the seasonings on hand. My family enjoys it with
steamed rice and sautéed broccoli. I have simmered sea scallops

and even a large whole grouper fillet in this flavorful sauce with spectacular results.

3 tablespoons nonfat yogurt

1 teaspoon sweet paprika

1 teaspoon garam masala (see Note)

1 tablespoon tomato paste

½ cup light coconut milk (I use A Taste of Thai, unsweetened)

½ teaspoon chili powder

Kosher salt

1 tablespoon peanut oil

2 garlic cloves, minced

1 teaspoon grated fresh peeled ginger

¼ teaspoon ground cinnamon

1 teaspoon cornstarch dissolved in 1 tablespoon coconut milk

1½ pounds large shrimp, peeled and deveined

2 tablespoons coarsely chopped cilantro

Freshly ground black pepper

Whisk together the yogurt, paprika, garam masala, tomato paste, coconut milk, chili powder, and ⅔ cup water in a small bowl, season with ½ teaspoon salt, and set aside. Heat the peanut oil in a deep nonstick skillet over medium heat and sauté the garlic, ginger, and cinnamon for 1 to 2 minutes, until fragrant. Add the yogurt mixture and bring to a boil, stirring occasionally, then lower the heat and simmer for 5 minutes to blend the flavors. Stir in the cornstarch mixture and cook until thick and smooth. Add the shrimp and simmer until the shrimp start to curl and are just cooked through, 2 to 3 minutes. Stir in the cilantro and season with salt and pepper.

Note: Garam masala is an Indian spice blend that may include black pepper, cardamom, cinnamon, cumin, and cloves.

Either the same day or the next day, I usually make the coconut custards on page 251 for dessert to use the remaining coconut milk from this recipe.

grilled shrimp
with romesco sauce

WLS ½ portion: Calories 149, fat 8 gr, carbs 3 gr, protein 16 gr
Serves 4

Creamy red pepper aioli—in this Spanish version with almonds, called *romesco*—is delicious with all types of grilled or roasted fish and chicken. This recipe makes about one cup of sauce, which is plenty for two meals. Pair the leftover sauce with grilled chicken thighs. Serve with roasted asparagus and a tomato salad dressed with balsamic vinegar and olive oil.

4 garlic cloves
½ medium onion, cut into ½-inch slices
¼ cup whole almonds
One 1-inch slice French bread, cubed
1 Roma tomato, cut in half lengthwise
3 tablespoons olive oil
¼ cup roasted red peppers, drained well and patted dry
1 tablespoon red wine vinegar
¼ teaspoon crushed red pepper flakes
1 teaspoon sweet paprika
Kosher salt and freshly ground black pepper
1½ pounds jumbo shrimp, peeled and butterflied

Preheat the oven to 400°F. Arrange the garlic, onion, almonds, bread, and tomato on a baking sheet, drizzle with 1 teaspoon of the olive oil, and roast for 12 to 15 minutes, until the vegetables are softened and the bread and almonds are golden. Transfer to a food processor and add the roasted peppers, vinegar, red pepper flakes, and paprika. Pulse until well combined, then slowly add the remaining olive oil, blending until the sauce is smooth and creamy. Season with salt and pepper.

Arrange the shrimp on small bamboo skewers and sear in a nonstick skillet or grill pan over high heat for 3 to 4 minutes, until just opaque throughout. Spoon a little of the sauce on each plate and arrange the shrimp around the sauce.

shrimp with roasted red onion and tomatillo salsa

WLS ½ portion: Calories 128, fat 5 gr, carbs 5 gr, protein 15 gr
Serves 4

Tomatillos look like green tomatoes, but they are related to the gooseberry. Popular in Latin-American cooking, tomatillos are the main ingredient in many green salsas or roasted salsa verde, lending a refreshing tartness. If you have never tasted them, give this recipe a try—they blend beautifully with the roasted red onion, jalapeños, garlic, and a touch of lime.

12 medium fresh tomatillos, husks removed, rinsed, and halved
2 fresh jalapeño chiles, halved lengthwise, stemmed, and seeded
4 garlic cloves
1 small red onion, cut into ½-inch slices
2 tablespoons olive oil
Kosher salt

2 tablespoons coarsely chopped cilantro
Juice of 1 lime, 1½ to 2 tablespoons
Freshly ground black pepper
1½ pounds large shrimp, peeled and deveined

Preheat the broiler. Arrange the tomatillos and jalapeños cut side down along with the garlic and onion slices on a baking sheet; drizzle with 1 tablespoon of the olive oil and sprinkle lightly with salt. Broil until the vegetables are charred on top and very soft, about 15 minutes. Empty the softened vegetables and any liquid into a food processor; pulse until chunky, then add the cilantro and process to a coarse puree. Transfer to a medium bowl, stir in the lime juice, and season with salt and pepper.

Heat the remaining tablespoon of olive oil over medium-high heat in a nonstick skillet and sauté the shrimp until they begin to turn pink. Add enough of the roasted red onion and tomatillo sauce to generously coat, and cook until the shrimp are just cooked through and the sauce is bubbling, about 4 minutes.

shrimp creole

WLS ½ portion: Calories 117, fat 3 gr, carbs 7 gr,
protein 15 gr
Serves 4

The traditional Louisiana favorite, a flavorful "trinity" of vegetables simmered in a tomato base and spiced up with Worcestershire, Tabasco, and a home-blended Creole seasoning. Use the biggest shrimp you can find and poach them in this delicious sauce just until they have firmed up and are opaque in the center. Serve the shrimp with a ladleful of sauce over some steamed rice for those who are not watching their carbohydrate count, with sautéed zucchini as a side dish.

½ cup chopped onion

½ cup chopped celery

½ cup diced green bell peppers

2 garlic cloves, chopped

1 tablespoon olive oil

One 16-ounce can diced tomatoes with juice

One 8-ounce can tomato sauce

1 tablespoon Worcestershire sauce

1 teaspoon Creole Seasoning Blend (recipe follows) or prepared Cajun or Creole blend

2 teaspoons Tabasco sauce, plus additional to taste

1 teaspoon cornstarch

Kosher salt and freshly ground black pepper

1½ pounds large shrimp, peeled and deveined

Sauté the onions, celery, peppers, and garlic in the olive oil in a non-stick skillet over medium heat until the vegetables are softened. Add the tomatoes, tomato sauce, Worcestershire sauce, Creole Seasoning, and Tabasco Sauce. Cover the pan, reduce the heat, and simmer for 45 minutes, or until the vegetables are tender. Blend the cornstarch with 1 tablespoon water, stir into the sauce, and cook until the mixture thickens. Season with salt, pepper, and additional Tabasco sauce to taste. Add the shrimp, cover, and simmer for 4 to 5 minutes, until the shrimp are pink and just cooked through.

creole seasoning blend

2½ tablespoons sweet paprika

2 tablespoons kosher salt

2 tablespoons garlic powder
1 tablespoon black pepper
1 tablespoon onion powder
1 tablespoon cayenne
1 tablespoon dried oregano
1 tablespoon dried thyme

Combine all the ingredients thoroughly and store in an airtight jar or container.

Note: If you'd rather use a prepared blend, Tony Chachere's makes several excellent Creole seasonings (see Sources, page 303).

shrimp ceviche

WLS ½ portion: Calories 166, fat 9 gr, carbs 6.5 gr,
protein 15.5 gr
Serves 4

When I lived in Mexico, nothing was tastier on a sunny afternoon than a ceviche cocktail, prepared with chunks of fresh snapper, conch, and shrimp, all "cooked" by the acid in the lime juice and tossed with tomatoes, onion, cilantro, and a touch of habanero. The little open-air seafood restaurants along the beach served these delicious salads piled in old-fashioned ice cream sundae glasses with half a lime and a basket of freshly fried tortilla chips. Here, the shrimp are briefly poached to make them tender.

Kosher salt and freshly ground black pepper
Juice of 4 limes (about ¾ cup), plus 1 lime cut into wedges
1¼ pounds medium shrimp, peeled and deveined

3 ripe Roma tomatoes, diced

1 small red onion, finely diced

1 jalapeño chile, stemmed, seeded, and very finely minced

½ cup green olive pieces

½ cup coarsely chopped cilantro

2 tablespoons olive oil

1 tablespoon ketchup

Tabasco sauce to taste

4 corn tortillas

1 small ripe Hass avocado, peeled and cut into 1-inch cubes

Fill a large saucepan halfway with water; add 1 tablespoon salt and the juice and rind of 1 lime (about 1½ tablespoons of juice) and bring to a boil over high heat. Add the shrimp, remove from the heat, and poach for 60 to 90 seconds. Drain the shrimp and then immediately rinse with cool water. Peel and devein the poached shrimp and place in a large bowl. Add the tomatoes, onion, jalapeño, olives, cilantro, olive oil, ketchup, lime juice, and Tabasco and combine to blend. Season with salt and pepper. Chill before serving.

Preheat the oven to 350°F. Cut the tortillas into eight wedges and spread out on a baking sheet; sprinkle with salt and bake for 10 to 15 minutes, until golden and crisp.

Serve a generous portion of the ceviche in a martini glass or decorative dish, garnishing with a few avocado cubes, a lime wedge, and baked tortilla chips.

Note: Avocados are ripe when they are almost black and yield slightly when pressed with your thumb.

southern shrimp and grits

WLS ½ portion: Calories 133, fat 6 gr, carbs 3 gr,
protein 16 gr
Serves 4

This version of the Low Country favorite is spicy, but you can tame it if you would like by cutting the seasoning in half and using less Tabasco. I buy my stone-ground grits from a mill in northern Georgia. My husband and his family can't believe an Italian from New Jersey can make such a delicious bowl of grits. I have my shrimp and sauce in a bowl and pass on the grits. The WLS portion does not include any grits in the nutritional analysis.

1¼ pounds large shrimp, peeled and deveined
1 teaspoon Creole Seasoning Blend, page 164, or prepared
    Creole or Cajun blend (see Note, page 165)
1½ teaspoons sweet paprika
Juice of 1 lemon, about 2 tablespoons
1 cup stone-ground white grits (see Note)
Kosher salt
1 tablespoon salted butter
½ cup shredded Cheddar, about ⅛ pound
2 teaspoons Tabasco sauce
Freshly ground black pepper
3 slices bacon, cut into 1-inch pieces
1 small onion, chopped
3 garlic cloves, thinly sliced
½ cup chopped green bell pepper
½ cup chicken broth (see Note, page 127)
2 teaspoons Worcestershire sauce

1 teaspoon cornstarch

4 green onions (scallions), thinly sliced

Toss the shrimp with the Creole seasoning, paprika, and lemon juice in a large bowl until evenly coated. Set aside.

Prepare the grits in a large heavy saucepan, first bringing 3 cups of water and 1 teaspoon of salt to a boil. Slowly whisk in the grits, cover, and reduce the heat to a very low simmer. Cook, stirring occasionally, for 25 to 30 minutes, until the grits are thick and creamy. Stir in the butter, cheese, and 1 teaspoon of the Tabasco, and season with salt and pepper. Set aside.

Brown the bacon in a nonstick skillet over medium-high heat and transfer to a paper towel to drain. Add the onion, garlic, and green pepper to the bacon fat in the skillet and cook until the vegetables are very tender, about 5 minutes. Add ¼ cup of the chicken broth, the Worcestershire, and the remaining teaspoon of Tabasco. In a separate bowl, blend the cornstarch with the remaining ¼ cup broth; add to the vegetables in the skillet. Cook, stirring constantly, until smooth and thick, about 2 minutes. Add the shrimp to the sauce and cook until they begin to curl and turn pink, about 2 minutes. Stir in the green onions and continue cooking until the shrimp are opaque throughout. Place a scoop of hot stone-ground grits in a deep bowl and cover with shrimp and sauce.

Note: The grits I order from the Nora Mill Granary are excellent.

almond shrimp cakes with
sesame chili mayonnaise

WLS 1 shrimp cake: Calories 126, fat 6 gr, carbs 4 gr,
protein 14 gr
Makes 8 cakes

This is a superb alternative to a crab cake or salmon patty, and it
goes together just as quickly. Use a small scoop to form bite-size
patties to serve as a first course or party food. These almond-
crusted cakes will remind you of shrimp toast!

½ cup mayonnaise
2 teaspoons soy sauce
2 teaspoons hot chili oil or sesame oil
1 bacon slice, chopped
1 pound raw shrimp, peeled and cleaned
1 slice whole wheat sandwich bread
¼ cup milk
4 green onions (scallions), sliced
2 teaspoons cornstarch
¾ teaspoon salt
¼ teaspoon freshly ground black pepper
2 cups sliced almonds
2 tablespoons vegetable oil

Blend the mayonnaise, soy sauce, and 1 teaspoon of the chili oil; set
aside.

Pulse the bacon in a food processor until finely chopped. Add the
shrimp to the bacon and pulse until the shrimp are coarsely chopped;
do not puree. Soak the bread in the milk in a small bowl, mash with

a fork, and add to the shrimp. Pulse until just combined. Transfer the shrimp mixture to a large bowl, then stir in the green onions, cornstarch, the remaining chili oil, salt, and pepper. Spread the almonds on a piece of plastic wrap and, using a ¼-cup measure or small ice-cream scoop, drop 1 mound of shrimp mixture onto the almonds. Sprinkle the top of the mound with almonds to coat and press to slightly flatten into a 3-inch cake. Repeat with the remaining mixture and almonds.

Heat 1 tablespoon of the vegetable oil in a nonstick skillet over medium-high heat and sauté the first 4 cakes, turning once, until golden brown on both sides. Remove to a plate and cover with foil. Cook the remaining cakes. Serve warm with a dab of sesame chili mayonnaise.

grilled shrimp with balsamic vegetable salad

WLS portion (3 ounces shrimp and ¼-cup vegetable salad):
Calories 235, fat 8 gr, carbs 5 gr, protein 23 gr
Serves 6

This is a simple but impressive meal for a weekend barbecue with friends. The lightly seasoned grilled shrimp are moistened by the grilled vegetable salad that gives this entrée an excellent texture. The grilled salad can be enhanced as well as made more substantial by tossing the finished dressed vegetables with a package of Near East brand roasted garlic or Parmesan couscous prepared according to the package directions. A steaming platter of freshly boiled corn is a wonderful addition to the table.

Vegetable oil cooking spray

⅔ cup olive oil

4 garlic cloves, minced

1 large red onion, cut into ½-inch slices

1 small eggplant, cut crosswise into ½-inch-thick rounds

2 red or yellow bell peppers, cut into quarters

2 small zucchini, cut in half lengthwise

4 jalapeño peppers, left whole

4 small or 2 large portobello mushrooms

Kosher salt and freshly ground black pepper

¼ cup chopped basil

3 tablespoons balsamic vinegar

2 pounds large shrimp, peeled with tails left on

Spray a grill with vegetable oil spray and preheat to high. Combine the olive oil with the garlic; brush the cut vegetables with 2 tablespoons of the flavored oil and season with salt and pepper. Arrange on the grill and cook until softened and beginning to char on the edges, 5 to 8 minutes. Remove to a large bowl and set aside. When the vegetables are cool enough to handle, cut them into 1-inch pieces and toss in a large salad bowl with ¼ cup of the garlic oil, the basil, and balsamic vinegar.

Baste the shrimp with garlic oil, season with salt and pepper, and grill until just cooked through, 2 to 3 minutes per side. Arrange on serving plates and spoon on some of the grilled vegetable salad.

seared scallop salad
with mustard dressing

WLS ½ portion: Calories 154, fat 9 gr, carbs 5 gr, protein 13.5 gr
Serves 4

I find that most people who have bariatric surgery crave green
vegetables in the two- to four-month range post-op, and this salad
is satisfying. Scallops are moist and tender as long as they are
seared until they are just cooked through. The tender spinach
leaves are low in carbohydrates. The dressing is tangy and
smooth. You can substitute shrimp or chunks of mahimahi for
the scallops.

6 cups baby spinach leaves, rinsed and dried
1 ripe Hass avocado, halved lengthwise and cut crosswise into
**   half-moon slices**
1½ pounds large sea scallops, tough tendons removed
1 tablespoon olive oil
Kosher salt and freshly ground black pepper
2 garlic cloves, minced
½ teaspoon sweet paprika
¼ cup sour cream
2 tablespoons light mayonnaise
1 tablespoon Dijon mustard
Juice of 1 lemon, about 2 tablespoons

Make a small bed of baby spinach leaves on 4 dinner plates and arrange the avocado slices on top.

Preheat a large nonstick skillet over high heat. In a large bowl,
toss the scallops with the olive oil, salt, pepper, garlic, and paprika.

Sear the scallops a total of 3 to 4 minutes, turning once, until they are just opaque in the center. Reserving any pan juices, place a portion of broiled scallops on each salad. In a small bowl, combine the reserved scallop juices with the sour cream, mayonnaise, mustard, lemon juice, and salt and pepper to taste. Drizzle the dressing over the salads and serve.

salmon bruschetta

WLS ½ portion: Calories 166, fat 10 gr, carbs 2 gr, protein 15 gr
Serves 4

This recipe takes a richly flavored bruschetta salad that would be delicious on a piece of garlic toast and features it to accentuate a piece of perfectly roasted salmon. For this dish, I love the taste of the giant Cerignola olives.

Four 5- to 6-ounce salmon fillets
Kosher salt and freshly ground black pepper
⅔ cup black olive pieces, Cerignola or Kalamata
    (see Note, page 138)
3 ripe Roma tomatoes, diced
½ small red onion, minced
3 tablespoons olive oil
1 tablespoon balsamic vinegar
1 tablespoon julienned basil
1 garlic clove, minced

Preheat the oven to 425°F. Arrange the fillets on a baking sheet, season with salt and pepper, and roast 8 to 10 minutes per 1 inch of thickness, until the fish is just opaque throughout.

Combine the olives, tomatoes, onion, olive oil, vinegar, basil, and garlic in a medium bowl. Place the roasted fillets in the center of each plate and heap with the bruschetta mixture.

salmon baked in salsa verde

WLS ½ portion: Calories 145, fat 7.5 gr, carbs 3 gr, protein 16 gr
Serves 4

This dish is commonplace in Mexico but is usually prepared with grouper or snapper. I love the color and flavor contrast using a piece of fresh wild salmon. The salsa verde keeps the fish extremely moist. I serve this beautiful dish with yellow rice and seasoned black beans.

Four 5- to 6-ounce salmon fillets
Kosher salt and freshly ground black pepper
2 garlic cloves
1 poblano chile, stemmed, seeded, and chopped
¾ cup chopped cilantro, lightly packed
¾ cup chopped flat-leaf parsley, lightly packed
6 green onions (scallions), sliced
1 tablespoon white vinegar
2 ripe Roma tomatoes, diced
½ teaspoon dried oregano
2 tablespoons olive oil

Preheat the oven to 425°F. Season the fish with salt and pepper and place in a shallow baking dish. Combine the garlic, chile, cilantro, parsley, green onions, vinegar, tomatoes, oregano, and olive oil in a blender or food processor and coarsely puree. Season with salt and pepper. Pour the salsa verde mixture over the fish and bake for 25 to 30 minutes, until the fish is opaque throughout. Carefully remove the fillets to serving plates and spoon some of the sauce over the top.

roasted salmon
with tzatziki sauce

WLS ½ portion: Calories 144, fat 7 gr, carbs 3 gr, protein 16 gr
Serves 4

This cool cucumber-garlic sauce is one of my favorites. It is perfect for a beautifully roasted piece of salmon; the garlic, tart yogurt, and cucumber are a classic combination. If you have any of the tzatziki left over, serve it with pita bread wedges that you have baked to a golden crisp in a 350°F oven. I will roast an entire side of salmon fillet, and use the leftovers for a fast and delicious lunch entrée. Just flake the cold salmon, toss it with some of the tzatziki sauce, and serve it over a bed of baby spinach leaves that have been dressed with a little olive oil and lemon juice.

1 medium cucumber, peeled and seeded
½ cup low-fat yogurt
2 tablespoons light mayonnaise
Juice of ½ lemon, about 1 tablespoon
4 garlic cloves, mashed to a paste with a little salt
3 green onions (scallions), thinly sliced, including tender green tops
2 tablespoons chopped fresh dill
Kosher salt and freshly ground black pepper
Four 5- to 6-ounce salmon fillets

Preheat the oven to 425°F. Grate the cucumber using the large holes on a box grater and squeeze to remove excess liquid. Place in a large bowl and combine with the yogurt, mayonnaise, lemon juice, garlic, green onions, and dill; add salt and plenty of black pepper. Arrange the fish on a baking sheet and season with salt and pepper. Roast for 8 to 10 minutes, until just opaque throughout. Transfer the fish to serving plates and spoon some of the tzatziki sauce on top.

salmon burgers with artichoke tartar sauce

WLS ½ portion: Calories 161, fat 10 gr, carbs 3 gr, protein 16 gr
Serves 4

This is a different but simple way to prepare heart-healthy salmon. I buy wild salmon whenever it is available, but as long as the farm-raised is impeccably fresh it is reliable and delicious. The artichoke tartar sauce is simply scrumptious; I also use it as a sauce for sautéed or grilled shrimp and scallops.

burgers

1¼ to 1½ pounds salmon fillet, trimmed of skin,
   with pin bones removed
2 tablespoons light mayonnaise
1 tablespoon chopped dill
½ teaspoon kosher salt
½ teaspoon freshly ground black pepper

sauce

> 4 whole canned artichoke hearts, well drained and finely diced
>
> ¼ cup light mayonnaise
>
> 1 tablespoon minced red onion
>
> 1 tablespoon small capers, rinsed, drained, and coarsely chopped
>
> 1 teaspoon fresh lemon juice
>
> 1 tablespoon minced sweet pickle (Mt. Olive Pickle Company
>   makes a no-sugar-added sweet gherkin using Splenda)
>
> 1 tablespoon chopped flat-leaf parsley
>
> Vegetable oil cooking spray

Coarsely grind the salmon in a food processor by pulsing on and off. Transfer to a bowl, fold in the mayonnaise, dill, salt, and pepper, and form into four ½-inch-thick patties. Cover and refrigerate for 1 hour to make the burgers easier to handle.

Mix the artichokes, mayonnaise, onion, capers, lemon juice, pickle, and parsley in a medium bowl until well combined; cover and chill until serving.

Preheat a lightly oiled nonstick skillet over medium-high heat. Sear the salmon burgers until the fish is just cooked through, 2 to 3 minutes per side. Place the burgers on plates and top with some of the sauce.

roasted salmon with mango salsa

WLS ½ portion: Calories 153, fat 8 gr, carbs 6 gr, protein 15 gr
Serves 4

Mango salsa is my all-time favorite. I love to combine the
sweetness of fresh fruit with savory flavors and citrus as an

before

accompaniment for fish, seafood, and meats. Mango is very juicy and makes the fish wonderfully moist. When the backyard mango trees in my area are heavy with fruit, my friends bring me shopping bags full in hopes of being rewarded with a big bowl of this salsa. A tiny piece of grilled salmon with a spoonful of mango salsa was one of my first soft food meals after my surgery. Roast a double portion of the salmon and use the leftovers to make a salmon-mango salad for the next day's lunch by flaking the cold fillet and combining with a few spoonfuls of the salsa.

1 large ripe mango
Juice of 2 limes, 3 to 4 tablespoons
½ cup chopped fresh cilantro
1 small red onion, minced
2 tablespoons plus 1 teaspoon extra-virgin olive oil
Kosher salt and freshly ground black pepper
Several pinches of ground chipotle chile or cayenne, or a few
**   dashes of Tabasco Chipotle sauce**
Four 5- to 6-ounce salmon fillets

Preheat the oven to 425°F.

Peel the skin from the mango, slice off each fleshy half parallel to the flat seed, and cut into even, ½-inch dice. Mix the diced mango with the lime juice, cilantro, onion, and 2 tablespoons of the oil, adding salt, pepper, and hot pepper to taste.

Rub the salmon with the remaining teaspoon of olive oil, arrange on a baking sheet, and season with salt and pepper. Roast for 8 to 10 minutes per 1 inch of thickness of salmon fillet, measuring at the thickest point. Transfer to plates and spoon on the mango salsa.

grilled salmon
with wasabi sauce

WLS ½ portion: Calories 150, fat 8 gr, carbs 2 gr, protein 16 gr
Serves 4

I am a serious fan of wasabi, the pungent green Japanese
horseradish. This quick sauce is sharp and creamy; a perfect
companion for the soy-sesame-glazed salmon fillet. Adjust the
amount of wasabi to your taste. This sauce is also delicious as
a dip for grilled skewered garlic shrimp or to drizzle over soy-
sesame-marinated chicken.

¾ **cup soy sauce**
1 tablespoon sesame oil
Four 5- to 6-ounce salmon fillets
1 tablespoon Japanese wasabi powder or 2 teaspoons prepared paste
¼ **cup reduced-fat sour cream**
2 tablespoons light mayonnaise (see Note, page 137)
Kosher salt and freshly ground black pepper
3 green onions (scallions), thinly sliced

Blend the soy sauce with the sesame oil and pour over the salmon in a
shallow dish. Marinate the salmon for 30 to 60 minutes.

In a small bowl, mix the wasabi powder with enough warm water
to make a smooth, thick paste. Whisk in the sour cream and mayonnaise, then season with salt and pepper to taste. Add a little water to
bring the mixture to a sauce consistency.

Preheat a grill pan or large nonstick skillet. Remove the fillets
from the marinade and pat dry with paper towels. Place the fillets in
the hot grill pan flesh-side down, and sear for 4 minutes. Carefully

before

turn and cook the fillets for an additional 4 minutes, or until just barely cooked throughout. Transfer to plates, drizzle with wasabi sauce, and sprinkle with the sliced scallions.

catfish with
spicy orange sauce

WLS ½ portion: Calories 140, fat 9 gr, carbs 4 gr, protein 11 gr
Serves 4

Catfish is a meaty, mild fish that is always available. This recipe pairs essential Asian flavors with orange juice, and can be put together in minutes while you dress some baby greens in the Sesame Dressing from page 219.

½ cup orange juice
1 tablespoon hoisin sauce, a sweet spicy Asian barbecue-style
 sauce, available in most supermarkets
2 tablespoons soy sauce
¼ cup sherry or Chinese cooking wine
1 teaspoon grated fresh ginger
1 garlic clove, minced
4 green onions (scallions), thinly sliced
2 teaspoons peanut oil
Four 5- to 6-ounce catfish fillets
All-purpose or Wondra flour for dusting

In a small bowl, blend the orange juice, hoisin sauce, soy sauce, and sherry; then stir in the ginger, garlic, and green onions. Heat the peanut oil over high heat in a large nonstick skillet or wok. Dry the fillets with paper towels and lightly dust with flour, patting off excess. Sear for 2 minutes, turn the fillets, and sear for 2 minutes more. Reduce the heat; add the sauce and simmer, covered, for 6 to 8 minutes, until the fish is opaque throughout. Transfer the fish to plates and spoon the sauce over.

roasted tilapia
with green chile crema

WLS ½ portion: Calories 97, fat 4 gr, carbs 2 gr, protein 18 gr
Serves 4

This simple sour cream–based sauce uses canned roasted green chiles and is delicious with a tilapia fillet. The sauce can be combined in minutes while the fish cooks, making this a perfect midweek meal. For your family, serve with yellow rice and seasoned black beans with garlic in olive oil.

Four 5- to 6-ounce tilapia fillets
1 teaspoon olive oil
Kosher salt and freshly ground black pepper
One 4-ounce can roasted mild green chiles, well drained, or
    ½ cup roasted salsa verde (see Note, page 131)
½ cup reduced-fat sour cream
¼ cup chopped cilantro
Juice of 1 lime, 1½ to 2 tablespoons

Preheat the oven to 425°F. Rub the fillets with the olive oil and season with salt and pepper. Roast for 6 to 8 minutes, until opaque throughout. Pulse the chiles, sour cream, cilantro, and lime juice in a food processor, and season with salt and pepper. Transfer the fish to plates and spoon on the green chile crema.

simple flounder with salsa

*WLS ½ portion: Calories 86, fat 3 gr, carbs 2 gr, protein 13 gr
Serves 4*

My easiest recipe! This one can be on the table in barely five minutes. Flounder fillets are very thin and can be sautéed in just a minute or two. Choose fillets that are 5 to 6 ounces each so you won't have to sauté more than one per person.

The taste of this finished dish varies with the kind of salsa you use. Try roasted garlic, fire-roasted tomato, tomatillo, or chipotle varieties. I am always on the lookout for unusual small-batch salsas to have on hand when I need to prepare a quick meal. Make sure you read the salsa label and avoid those with black beans, peaches, corn, and sweeteners, or you will unnecessarily increase your carbohydrate count. This simple preparation also works with tilapia, shrimp, scallops, or any sautéed fillet.

**Four 5- to 6-ounce flounder fillets; if fillets are smaller,
    serve 2 per person**
Kosher salt and freshly ground black pepper
All-purpose or Wondra flour for dusting
1 tablespoon olive oil
1 garlic clove, slivered
1 cup prepared salsa (see Note, page 131)
Juice of 1 lime, 1½ to 2 tablespoons
1 tablespoon chopped cilantro or flat-leaf parsley

Season the fillets with salt and pepper; lightly dust with flour and pat off any excess. Heat the oil in a nonstick skillet over medium-high heat; sauté the fillets for 2 minutes, carefully turn, cook for an additional minute or until just opaque throughout, and transfer to plates. Add the garlic to the skillet; sauté for 1 minute, or until lightly browned. Add the salsa, lime juice, and cilantro to the skillet and cook until bubbling and hot. Pour the sauce over the fish fillets, and serve immediately.

roasted grouper with tomatoes and herbed cream sauce

WLS ½ portion: Calories 134, fat 6.6 gr, carbs 6 gr, protein 16 gr
Serves 4

Grouper is usually available where I live in Florida, but feel free to substitute tilapia, snapper, or salmon if it is the better choice in your area. This is a very attractive dish with a colorful contrast between the cream sauce and the marinated tomato topping, and it would be an excellent meal for company served with couscous and sautéed zucchini slices.

2 large shallots, minced
Juice of 2 lemons, about ¼ cup
1 tablespoon white wine vinegar
1 cup evaporated low-fat milk
2 teaspoons minced fresh thyme
Kosher salt and freshly ground black pepper
2 ripe Roma tomatoes, finely diced

2 tablespoons olive oil

1 tablespoon julienned fresh basil

Four 5- to 6-ounce grouper fillets

Preheat the oven to 425°F.

Combine half of the shallots, 2 tablespoons of the lemon juice, and the vinegar in a small saucepan. Boil over medium-high heat until the liquid is reduced to a glaze, about 4 minutes. Add the milk and thyme, bring the mixture to a boil, reduce the heat, and simmer for 4 to 5 minutes, until thickened to a sauce consistency. Season with salt and pepper and set aside.

Combine the tomatoes, oil, and basil with the remaining shallots and lemon juice in a small bowl. Season with salt and pepper and set aside.

Season the fish with salt and pepper and arrange on a baking sheet. Roast for 8 to 10 minutes per inch of thickness, until the fish is opaque throughout. Transfer the fillets to serving plates. Spoon the warm cream sauce around the fish and mound some of the tomato mixture on top of each fillet.

grouper with red pepper coulis

WLS ½ portion: Calories 76, fat <1 gr, carbs 3 gr, protein 14 gr
Serves 4

This sauce has a wonderful Asian flavor that accents the sweetness of the red pepper and highlights a simply prepared piece of fish. Grouper is delicious, but buy whatever is freshest at your fish market; swordfish, salmon, flounder, shrimp, or scallops would be perfect when simply seasoned, grilled, and placed in a pool of this snappy red sauce. This meal can be completed with jasmine or basmati rice and snow peas that are quickly stir-fried in a teaspoon of peanut oil with garlic slivers.

2 red bell peppers, quartered, stems and seeds removed
½ medium onion, sliced
1 tablespoon grated fresh ginger
1 teaspoon Tabasco sauce
1 tablespoon rice wine vinegar
Kosher salt and freshly ground black pepper
Vegetable oil cooking spray
Four 5- to 6-ounce grouper fillets

Combine the peppers, onion, and ginger with ¾ cup water in a medium saucepan and bring to a boil. Reduce the heat, cover, and simmer until the peppers are very soft, about 12 minutes. Remove the peppers and onion with a slotted spoon and puree in a food processor. Blend in the Tabasco and vinegar, and season with salt and pepper.

Preheat the broiler or a lightly sprayed nonstick grill pan. Broil the grouper for no more than 10 minutes per inch of thickness, or grill in a grill pan, until just opaque throughout. Spoon a puddle of pepper puree on each plate and center a fish fillet on top of the sauce.

mahimahi with puttanesca sauce

WLS ½ portion: Calories 100, fat 3 gr, carbs 5 gr, protein 14 gr
Serves 4

This is a wonderful sauce for any firm, meaty fish, including grouper and swordfish. Do not shy away from this classic sauce because of the anchovies—they melt into the sauce and add a

mellow saltiness that cannot be duplicated. Serve with a mixed
tossed salad dressed with balsamic vinegar and olive oil.

1 tablespoon olive oil

2 garlic cloves, minced

1 medium red onion, thinly sliced

4 anchovy fillets, rinsed and minced

One 14-ounce can diced tomatoes, drained

⅓ cup oil-cured black Kalamata olive pieces (see Note, page 138)

2 tablespoons small capers, rinsed

1 teaspoon finely chopped fresh rosemary

Kosher salt and freshly ground black pepper

Four 5- to 6-ounce mahimahi pieces, cut 1 inch thick,
**   with skin removed**

⅓ cup chopped flat-leaf parsley

Pinch of crushed red pepper flakes

Preheat the oven to 425°F. Heat the olive oil in a medium saucepan
over medium-high heat and sauté the garlic and onion until softened,
about 4 minutes. Add the anchovies and cook until they have softened to a paste, about 2 minutes. Stir in the tomatoes, olives, capers,
and rosemary. Bring the sauce to a boil, reduce the heat, and simmer
for 5 minutes. Add salt and pepper to taste.

Arrange the fish pieces on a baking sheet and season with salt and
pepper. Roast the fish for 8 to 10 minutes, until just cooked through.
Place a piece of fish in the center of each plate. Stir the parsley and
red pepper flakes into the sauce and spoon over the fish.

swordfish with
charred tomato vinaigrette

WLS ½ portion: Calories 181, fat 10 gr, carbs 3 gr, protein 18 gr
Serves 4

Swordfish is my favorite fish. My local fish market sells its
swordfish steaks trimmed into 4- to 6-ounce serving pieces
with the tough skin and darker center flesh removed, which
makes the preparation even easier. The tomato vinaigrette from
this recipe is perfect with any broiled or grilled fish or shellfish;
the roasted tomato flavor is fantastic when paired with skewers of
grilled shrimp. Or use it on roasted and thinly sliced turkey breast.

4 large ripe Roma tomatoes, cut in half lengthwise
1 small red onion, sliced
3 garlic cloves, left whole
1 teaspoon chopped basil
1 teaspoon chopped thyme
1½ tablespoons balsamic vinegar
¼ cup extra-virgin olive oil
Kosher salt and freshly ground black pepper
Four 5- to 6-ounce swordfish pieces, cut 1 inch thick, trimmed
    with skin removed

Preheat the broiler. Arrange the tomatoes cut side down along with
the onion slices and garlic on a baking sheet. Broil for 12 to 15 minutes, until the tops of the vegetables are charred and the juices are
released. Remove from the broiler and pour the contents of the pan,
including juices, into a food processor; add the basil and thyme and
pulse until the sauce is blended but still has some texture. Transfer

the mixture to a bowl, stir in the vinegar and olive oil, and add salt and pepper to taste.

Season the fish with salt and pepper and broil for 8 to 10 minutes, until the fish is opaque throughout. Transfer the fish pieces to plates and spoon the charred tomato vinaigrette over the swordfish.

swordfish steaks
with cilantro cream

WLS ½ portion: Calories 145, fat 5.5 gr, carbs 3 gr, protein 20 gr
Serves 4

The cilantro cream is the star of this meal, making a piece of impeccably fresh grilled fish into something extraordinary. I wouldn't hesitate to substitute tilapia, grouper, flounder, jumbo shrimp, or sea scallops. For the others in your family, serve with saffron rice and ripe tomato slices.

1 teaspoon olive oil
2 large shallots, sliced
4 garlic cloves, sliced
⅔ cup chopped cilantro, lightly packed
½ cup chicken broth (see Note, page 127)
½ cup evaporated low-fat milk
Kosher salt and freshly ground black pepper
Four 5- to 6-ounce swordfish pieces, cut about 1 inch thick,
    trimmed of skin

Heat the olive oil in a small saucepan over medium-high heat and sauté the shallots and garlic until softened. Add the cilantro and toss for

15 seconds. Stir in the broth and milk, and cook for 1 minute to steep the herbs. Transfer the mixture to a blender and, tightly holding the lid with a kitchen towel, blend until the sauce is smooth. Return the sauce to the pan, bring to a boil, reduce the heat, and simmer, stirring occasionally, until it begins to thicken. Season to taste with salt and pepper, and set aside. Preheat the broiler or a grill pan. Cook the swordfish 5 to 6 minutes per side, until cooked throughout. Spoon some of the sauce on each plate and place a swordfish piece in the center.

Swordfish with Tarragon Cream

Substitute ⅓ cup fresh tarragon leaves for the cilantro and use a squeeze of fresh orange juice to season the fish.

sweet and sour fish

WLS ½ portion: Calories 105, fat 2 gr, carbs 4.5 gr, protein 15 gr
Serves 4

I get many requests to re-create this dish in a healthy fresh style that is weight-loss friendly, and this version is both. Once you master the snappy sauce, get creative and spoon it over grilled or roasted chicken, shrimp, or salmon, or even store-bought rotisserie chicken. This recipe makes enough sauce for you to divide and use for another meal; the sauce keeps, covered and chilled, for a week.

Four 6-ounce tilapia fillets
Kosher salt and freshly ground black pepper
One 20-ounce can Libby's Splenda-sweetened pineapple chunks
1 teaspoon cornstarch
1 medium onion, diced
2 garlic cloves, chopped

1 teaspoon vegetable oil
1 tablespoon soy sauce
1 tablespoon ketchup
1 tablespoon vinegar
One 12-ounce jar roasted red bell peppers, drained and diced
3 green onions (scallions), thinly sliced

Preheat the oven to 400°F. Arrange the fish fillets on a baking sheet and season with salt and pepper.

Drain the pineapple, reserving the juice in a small bowl. Blend 2 tablespoons of the reserved pineapple juice with the cornstarch and set aside. Sauté the onion and garlic in the oil over medium heat in a medium saucepan until very soft, 7 to 8 minutes. Add the remaining pineapple juice, the soy sauce, ketchup, and vinegar, and then stir in the roasted peppers. Increase the heat to medium high and when the mixture begins to bubble, slowly add the cornstarch mixture and cook, stirring constantly, until thickened and glossy. Reduce the heat to low, add the pineapple chunks and green onions, and simmer for 10 minutes; season with salt and pepper.

Roast the tilapia fillets for 6 to 8 minutes, until opaque throughout. Transfer to serving plates and spoon on some of the sauce. Use the remaining sauce for another meal.

roasted tilapia with fresh herbs

WLS ½ portion: Calories 139, fat 3 gr, carbs 1 gr, protein 20 gr
Serves 4

Tilapia is a very mild and tender farm-raised fish available
almost everywhere. You can use different fresh herbs for variety.

I love cilantro, dill, flat-leaf parsley, and basil. Don't be scared
to prepare fish; this is a good place to start. Serve with a green
salad or with halved grape tomatoes tossed with bottled dressing.

Four 6-ounce tilapia fillets
3 tablespoons reduced-fat mayonnaise
Kosher salt and freshly ground black pepper
½ cup finely chopped flat-leaf parsley
2 tablespoons finely chopped dill

Preheat the oven to 400°F. Place the fillets on a baking sheet or in a
roasting pan. Evenly spread a little of the mayonnaise over each fillet,
using the back of a spoon. Season the fillets with salt and pepper,
then sprinkle with the chopped herbs. Bake for 8 to 10 minutes, just
until opaque throughout.

halibut with
ginger-tahini sauce

WLS ½ portion: Calories 134.5, fat 7 gr, carbs 2 gr, protein 15 gr
Serves 4

I keep a jar of sesame paste—tahini—in my refrigerator to use
for hummus, and I wanted to find another use for this toasty nut
butter. This vinaigrette combines the distinctive Asian flavors
of sesame, pickled ginger, soy sauce, and green onion. For your
family, pair this with steamed rice and some roasted asparagus
spears. I can find jars of pickled ginger in my local supermarket;
however, the ginger at my local sushi bar tastes much better.
When we go for sushi, I ask the chef for a small plastic to-go cup

and he is always happy to oblige. You can substitute salmon or
swordfish.

1 teaspoon whole cumin seeds

2 tablespoons peanut oil

1 garlic clove, minced

2 tablespoons tahini (sesame paste)

1 tablespoon soy sauce

Juice of 2 limes, 3 to 4 tablespoons

2 green onions (scallions), thinly sliced

¼ cup finely chopped pickled ginger, also called *gari*

Kosher salt and freshly ground black pepper

Four 5- to 6-ounce halibut pieces, cut 1 inch thick, trimmed with
     skin removed

Toast the cumin seeds in a dry skillet over medium-high heat, moving the pan constantly, until they are fragrant. Transfer the cumin
seeds to a large bowl. Whisk in the peanut oil, garlic, tahini, soy
sauce, lime juice, and 3 tablespoons water, then stir in the green
onions and ginger. Season with salt and pepper. Marinate the fish for
30 to 45 minutes in ¼ cup of the marinade.

Preheat the oven to 425°F. Shake the marinade from the fish
pieces. Arrange the fish on a baking sheet and roast for 8 to 10 minutes, until cooked through but still moist. Serve the fish with a little of
the remaining ginger-tahini mixture as a sauce.

spiced tuna steaks with
fennel and red pepper sauté

WLS ½ portion: Calories 113, fat 3 gr, carbs 4 gr, protein 18 gr
Serves 4

A seared, meaty tuna steak with a fennel-and-black-pepper
crust is accompanied by a sautéed fennel and sweet red pepper
condiment. Do not overcook the tuna; just a minute of additional
heat can turn a delectable moist ruby-colored tuna fillet into a dry
brown hockey puck.

Four 5- to 6-ounce tuna steaks, cut 1 inch thick
1 tablespoon plus 1 teaspoon olive oil, plus extra for coating the
tuna
1 tablespoon whole fennel seeds
1½ teaspoons whole black peppercorns
1 medium fennel bulb, trimmed, cut into quarters, cored, and
thinly sliced lengthwise
1 medium red bell pepper, cut into quarters and thinly sliced
2 garlic cloves, sliced
1 tablespoon fresh lemon juice (about ½ lemon)
Kosher salt and freshly ground black pepper

Lightly rub one side of each piece of tuna with the oil. Crush the fennel seeds and peppercorns with the bottom of a small heavy skillet on
a cutting board; press some of the coarse mixture onto the oiled side
of each tuna steak and set aside. Heat 1 tablespoon of the olive oil in
a skillet over medium-high heat. Sauté the fennel, bell pepper, and
garlic, stirring occasionally, until lightly browned, about 4 minutes.
Add ¼ cup water, cover, reduce the heat, and simmer the vegetables

for 10 minutes, until the fennel is very tender. Uncover and boil until the liquid is nearly evaporated. Stir in the lemon juice, season with salt and pepper, and remove from the heat.

Heat the teaspoon of olive oil in a large nonstick skillet over high heat just until it begins to smoke. Add the tuna steaks spice side down, and sear, undisturbed, for 30 seconds; reduce the heat to medium-high and continue to cook for 1½ minutes. Carefully turn and sear the second side for an additional 1½ minutes. Remove the tuna steaks to a cutting board, and immediately cut each piece across the grain into ½-inch-thick slices. The tuna should be rare to medium-rare in the center. Fan the tuna pieces on each plate and spoon some of the fennel–bell pepper mixture on the side.

seafood fra diavola

WLS ½ portion: Calories 155, fat 8 gr, carbs 4 gr, protein 14 gr
Serves 4

When we traveled to San Francisco for the bariatric surgeons' convention, we sampled lots of fresh local seafood served simmered in traditional tomato-based sauces such as this one. You can use mussels and shrimp as I have chosen for this version, or create your own favorite, using scallops, crab, or even a whole fish fillet or cubes of a firm fish such as swordfish or mahimahi. I serve this delectable seafood and sauce in a deep bowl with a sprinkle of flat-leaf parsley and plenty of crusty sourdough for the family.

12 garlic cloves, chopped (about ⅓ cup)
1 teaspoon crushed red pepper flakes
¼ cup olive oil

One 28-ounce can whole tomatoes in puree

2 tablespoons tomato paste

½ teaspoon dried oregano

2 teaspoons dried basil

1 cup white wine or chicken broth (see Note, page 127)

½ cup pitted Kalamata or other black brine-cured olives

Kosher salt and freshly ground black pepper

1 pound mussels

1 pound large shrimp, peeled, deveined, and rinsed

Cook the garlic and red pepper flakes in the oil in a deep, heavy skillet over medium heat, stirring, until fragrant but not browned, about 2 minutes. Add the tomatoes with puree, tomato paste, oregano, basil, wine, and olives. Simmer uncovered, stirring occasionally and breaking up the tomatoes, for 15 to 20 minutes, until the sauce is thickened. Season with salt and pepper.

Just before serving, increase the heat under the sauce to medium high, add the mussels and shrimp, cover, and cook until the mussels are open wide, checking frequently after 3 minutes. (Discard any mussels that remain unopened after 6 minutes.) Serve immediately.

chicken and turkey

Chicken and turkey are excellent sources of protein. One boneless, skinless chicken thigh weighs approximately 2½ ounces and provides approximately 18 grams of lean protein. Of course, breast meat has fewer grams of fat, but it is drier in texture and is therefore more difficult to eat during those first post-op months. Turkey is even a little higher in protein content with 2½ ounces containing more than 20 grams of protein. Cornish game hens are super-moist when marinated, have very tender meat, and can be substituted for the chicken and turkey in several of the roasted recipes.

With all the problems people say they have with eating chicken in their early post-surgery months, you might wonder why a chapter on poultry is included. Having trouble eating certain foods is largely due to the texture of a dish and this, of course, has a great deal to do with how the food is cooked. When I ask my weight-loss surgery friends how the offending chicken was prepared, it was usually white meat, baked, broiled, or fried, and served plain. Aha! Chicken thighs are very moist and much easier to digest than breasts, so many of the recipes here use either boneless or whole thighs. I almost always use chicken thighs at home as my first choice, and I only started cooking breasts again eighteen months post-op. I still occasionally have a tough time eating chicken breasts; I have tried marinating them, poaching them, and saucing them, but they are just too dense in

consistency—I can only eat a few bites before I have an uncomfortable feeling of fullness and indigestion.

Consider the consistency of a bite of oven-baked chicken breast;
then think about the texture of chicken cacciatore, the chicken thighs
simmered in tomato sauce until tender. Which would you choose?

An instant-read thermometer is inexpensive, and indispensable.
You will marvel at how juicy a boneless roasted turkey breast really
is when it is perfectly cooked to an internal temperature of 160°F.
Roast a whole chicken, turkey, or game hen until the thickest part of
the thigh is cooked to an internal temperature of 170°F. I now buy
organic chicken parts; I can buy exactly the amount I like. I also prefer that the chickens are fed an organic diet with no antibiotics. They
are tastier than the supermarket chicken, and with the small portions
we eat post-op, quality is important.

These recipes serve four people who have not had gastric bypass
surgery. The person who is eating after having had bypass surgery
would be eating about half of one serving. For example, a recipe
using 8 large chicken thighs would feed 4 people, serving two thighs
per person; the WLS half portion would be one thigh with enough of
the sauce to moisten it. The nutritional analysis has been calculated
for the WLS half portion, including the sauce for that dish.

chicken cutlets with sun-dried
tomato dijon sauce

WLS ½ portion: Calories 119, fat 6 gr, carbs 3 gr, protein 15.5 gr
Serves 4

Pounding the chicken cutlets tenderizes them. I buy whole
boneless breasts, which I split horizontally with a sharp knife to

butterfly, and then pound between sheets of plastic wrap or wax paper. If you don't have a meat mallet, use a small, heavy pot or a rolling pin. I serve this to family with a side dish of spinach sautéed with garlic in olive oil, and Yukon gold mashed potatoes.

4 boneless, skinless chicken breast halves, about 1½ pounds
Kosher salt and freshly ground black pepper
All-purpose or Wondra flour for dusting
2 tablespoons olive oil
2 garlic cloves, thinly sliced
¼ cup finely diced sun-dried tomatoes, about 6 pieces
2 tablespoons Dijon mustard
½ cup evaporated low-fat milk
½ cup low-sodium chicken broth

Butterfly the chicken breast halves, and then pound to an even ½-inch thickness. Season the chicken with salt and pepper and dust very lightly with flour. Heat the olive oil in a large nonstick skillet over medium-high heat and sauté the chicken cutlets until browned on both sides and cooked through, about 2 minutes per side. Transfer them to a serving platter.

In the oil remaining in the skillet, sauté the garlic until softened, about 2 minutes. Reduce the heat to low; add the sun-dried tomatoes and mustard, and whisk in the evaporated milk and broth. Heat gently until the sauce thickens, stirring constantly, adding the accumulated juices from the chicken platter. Do not boil the sauce or it will separate.

Return the chicken cutlets to the pan and turn to coat with the sauce. Season with salt and pepper and serve immediately.

roasted chicken chipotle salad

WLS ½ portion: Calories 147, fat 3 gr, carbs <1 gr, protein 14 gr
Serves 4

A perfect salad for a lunch with my girlfriends! I started eating salad early after my surgery—the leaves are tender and the dressing makes them very moist. Eat the chicken first, and when you start getting full, nibble on a few shreds of lettuce and pieces of avocado. The blue corn tortilla crisps add just enough crunch along with a beautiful color contrast, but if you cannot find the blue tortillas, substitute white or yellow. I arrange this salad in a large bowl, then add the dressing at the last minute and toss to coat at the table; I divide the salad among individual plates and top each with a few of the blue corn tortilla shreds.

4 large chicken breast halves, about 2 pounds
Kosher salt and freshly ground black pepper
½ teaspoon chili powder (I use pure ground chipotle)
¼ cup light or reduced-fat mayonnaise
Juice of 1 lime, 1½ to 2 tablespoons
3 canned chipotle chiles in adobo sauce, scraped of seeds and
finely minced
1 garlic clove, minced
2 tablespoons chopped cilantro
Chicken broth, optional
1 large head romaine lettuce, torn into small pieces or
shredded
1 ripe Hass avocado, peeled and cut into 1-inch cubes
½ cup grape tomatoes, cut in half

**2 blue corn tortillas, cut into ¼-inch strips, salted, and baked at
350°F until crisp**

Preheat the oven to 400°F. Loosen the skin from the chicken but do
not remove. Season the meat with salt, pepper, and chili powder,
place on a baking sheet, and roast for 35 to 40 minutes, until the
juices run clear when the meat is pierced with the tip of a knife or
an instant-read thermometer registers 160°F. Set aside. When the
chicken is cool enough to handle, remove the skin and bones and pull
the meat apart into large pieces. Puree the mayonnaise, lime juice,
chipotles, garlic, and cilantro in a blender or food processor, adding
a little water or chicken broth for a slightly thinner consistency. Season with salt and pepper.

Arrange the lettuce, avocado, and tomatoes on plates; add some
of the shredded chicken, drizzle with the chipotle dressing, and pile
on a few crisp tortilla pieces.

jerk chicken with
black bean and red pepper sauté

WLS ½ portion: Calories 151, fat 6 gr, carbs 9 gr, protein 16 gr
Serves 4

We have traveled to the islands of the Caribbean throughout the
years, which has given me the chance to sample jerk marinades
in numerous locations. I love the contrasts of the citrus, herbs,
and spices in this Jamaican dish. This dish requires advance
preparation.

4 large chicken breast halves, about 2 pounds
4 green onions (scallions), thinly sliced

3 garlic cloves, crushed

3 jalapeño chiles, stemmed, seeded, and minced

Juice of 2 limes, 3 to 4 tablespoons

Juice of 1 orange, about ⅓ cup

2 tablespoons chopped fresh thyme or 2 teaspoons dried thyme

3 tablespoons olive oil

¼ teaspoon freshly ground black pepper, plus additional to taste

½ teaspoon cayenne

½ teaspoon ground cinnamon

¼ teaspoon ground allspice

1 red bell pepper, diced

1 small red onion, diced

One 15-ounce can black beans, rinsed and drained

½ cup chicken broth (see Note, page 127)

Kosher salt

Loosen the skin on the chicken breasts but do not remove. Place the green onions, 2 of the garlic cloves, 2 of the jalapeños, the juice of 1 lime (1½ to 2 tablespoons), orange juice, thyme, 2 tablespoons of the olive oil, the pepper, cayenne, cinnamon, and allspice in a food processor and pulse to combine. Pour the jerk marinade over the chicken in a deep bowl or plastic bag, and refrigerate for 4 to 24 hours.

Preheat the oven to 425°F. Drain the chicken; arrange the pieces on a baking sheet and roast for 30 to 35 minutes, until the juices run clear when the meat is pierced with the tip of a knife or an instant-read thermometer registers 160°F.

Heat the remaining tablespoon of olive oil in a medium skillet over medium-high heat and sauté the remaining jalapeño and garlic clove, along with the bell pepper and onion, until lightly browned and softened, about 5 minutes. Stir in the beans, the remaining lime juice, and the chicken broth, slightly mashing the vegetables together. Reduce the heat and simmer for 15 minutes. Season with salt and pepper.

When the chicken is cool enough to handle, remove the skin and bones and cut into thick slices. To serve, spoon some of the black bean and red pepper sauté on a plate and arrange the chicken slices on top.

chicken marsala

WLS ½ portion: Calories 114, fat 4 gr, carbs 2 gr, protein 15 gr
Serves 4

Serve this to family over a pile of thin spaghetti dressed with a little olive oil, salt, pepper, red pepper flakes, and parsley; steamed broccoli adds low-carbohydrate nutrition and color.

4 boneless, skinless chicken breast halves, about 1½ pounds

Kosher salt and freshly ground black pepper

All-purpose or Wondra flour for dusting

1 tablespoon olive oil

1 tablespoon salted butter

1 small onion, finely diced

8 ounces cremini or button mushrooms, sliced

½ cup Marsala wine

½ cup low-sodium chicken broth

1 teaspoon cornstarch dissolved in 1 tablespoon water

2 tablespoons chopped flat-leaf parsley

Butterfly the chicken breast halves, and pound to an even ½-inch thickness. Season the chicken with salt and pepper and dust lightly with flour. Heat the olive oil in a large nonstick skillet over medium-high heat and sauté the chicken cutlets until lightly browned on both sides, about 2 minutes per side; transfer to a serving platter when finished. Add the butter to the oil remaining in the pan, and sauté the onion and mushrooms until the liquid has evaporated and the mushrooms start to brown, about 4 minutes. Add the wine, chicken broth, and the chicken with any accumulated juices from the platter, and simmer for 3 to 4 minutes, until the chicken is cooked through. Transfer the chicken back to the serving platter; thicken the sauce with the cornstarch mixture. Stir in the parsley and pour the sauce over the chicken.

chicken with dijon-orange sauce

WLS ½ portion: Calories 91, fat 3 gr, carbs 2.5 gr, protein 14 gr
Serves 4

Tender chicken cutlets with a sweet and sharp sauce can be quickly prepared and on the table in just 15 minutes. They pair perfectly with a simple tossed salad with balsamic vinaigrette and spinach sautéed in olive oil with garlic.

4 boneless, skinless chicken breast halves, about 1½ pounds
Kosher salt and freshly ground black pepper
All-purpose or Wondra flour for dusting
1 tablespoon olive oil
1 garlic clove, minced
½ cup orange juice
2 tablespoons Dijon mustard
2 tablespoons Nature's Hollow Apricot Preserves
½ teaspoon Tabasco sauce
2 green onions (scallions), thinly sliced

Butterfly the chicken breast halves, and pound to an even ½-inch thickness. Season the chicken with salt and pepper and dust lightly with flour. Heat the olive oil in a large nonstick skillet over medium-high heat and sauté the chicken cutlets until lightly browned on both sides and cooked through, about 2 minutes per side; transfer to a serving platter. Sauté the garlic in the oil remaining in the pan for 1 minute; stir in the orange juice, mustard, preserves, Tabasco, and green onions. Bring to a boil and cook until the sauce has thickened, about 4 minutes. Return the chicken to the skillet, coat with sauce, and simmer until heated through.

pollo acapulco
(chicken simmered in ancho-
guajillo sauce)

WLS ½ portion: Calories 127, fat 5 gr, carbs 6 gr, protein 14.5 gr
Serves 4

This recipe was inspired by several large bags of dried chiles, in shades of red from vermilion to mahogany, brought home from a Mexican vacation. It is delicious with various combinations of dried peppers, but try to use some of the sweeter varieties; this dish is about flavor, not heat. I have made the dish with only ancho chiles and have even added a few dried chipotles for different but equally delicious results. The texture of the simmered chicken is very easy for people to eat early after bariatric surgery. This makes a perfect meal for my family served with herbed rice and a salad.

3 dried ancho chiles (see Sources, page 303)

3 dried guajillo chiles (see Sources, page 303)

2 tablespoons olive oil

1 large sweet onion, chopped

5 garlic cloves, sliced

One 14-ounce can diced tomatoes, drained (see Note, page 148)

8 large bone-in, skinless chicken thighs, about 2 pounds

Kosher salt and freshly ground black pepper

½ cup chopped cilantro

Tear the dried chiles into large flat pieces, removing and discarding the stems and seeds. Toast the chile pieces for a few seconds, one at a time, in a nonstick skillet over medium-high heat, pressing down with a spatula until slight wisps of smoke appear. Transfer the toasted chiles to a small deep bowl, cover with 1 cup of very hot water to soften, and set aside while preparing the remaining ingredients.

Heat 1 tablespoon of the olive oil in a skillet over medium-high heat and sauté the onion and garlic until lightly browned and softened, about 5 minutes. Add the tomatoes, bring to a boil, reduce the heat, and simmer for 5 minutes. Place the drained chiles and the tomato-onion mixture in a blender, and puree until very smooth. Set aside. (Be careful when blending hot liquids: always tightly hold down the lid with a kitchen towel, because the hot liquids will expand the container when blended; it is safest to pulse the mixture.)

Season the chicken pieces with salt and pepper and brown in a nonstick skillet with the remaining tablespoon of olive oil over medium-high heat; drain any accumulated fat. Add the pureed sauce, cover the skillet, lower the heat, and simmer for 45 minutes, or until the chicken is very tender. Transfer the chicken pieces to a platter. Stir the cilantro into the sauce, season with salt and pepper, and pour over the chicken.

Ancho-Guajillo Shrimp

This recipe makes enough sauce that I can set a generous cup aside and save it for a shrimp meal later in the week. I sauté a little chopped garlic in some olive oil, then add the reserved ancho-guajillo sauce and simmer for 20 minutes to smooth out the flavors; add 1¼ pounds of peeled and deveined shrimp and cook until the shrimp are just opaque, adding a handful of chopped cilantro just before serving.

baja roasted chicken
with spicy avocado crema

WLS ½ portion: Calories 131, fat 7 gr, carbs 3 gr, protein 14.5 gr
Serves 4

I love to use spice rubs on roasted meats. I serve this entrée with saffron rice and a simple cherry tomato salad dressed with lime juice and olive oil. Any extra Spicy Avocado Crema can be enjoyed with tortilla chips.

1 tablespoon chopped cilantro

1 teaspoon poultry seasoning

1 teaspoon garlic powder

½ teaspoon sweet paprika

½ teaspoon kosher salt

½ teaspoon coarsely ground black pepper

¼ teaspoon crushed red pepper flakes

1 tablespoon olive oil

8 large boneless, skinless chicken thighs, about 1½ pounds

spicy avocado crema

>   1 large ripe Hass avocado, peeled and cut into chunks
>
>   2 garlic cloves, sliced
>
>   2 green onions (scallions), sliced
>
>   2 tablespoons chopped cilantro
>
>   ¼ cup reduced-fat sour cream
>
>   Juice of 1 lime, 1½ to 2 tablespoons
>
>   Few dashes of Tabasco sauce
>
>   About ¼ cup low-sodium chicken broth
>
>   Kosher salt and freshly ground black pepper

Preheat the oven to 400°F. Combine the cilantro, poultry season-ing, garlic powder, paprika, salt, black pepper, red pepper flakes, and olive oil in a small bowl, blending to form a paste. Rub a little of the mixture on each chicken thigh and arrange the thighs in a me-dium roasting pan. Roast without turning for 35 minutes, or until the chicken is golden brown and fork-tender.

Puree the avocado, garlic, green onions, and cilantro in a food processor. Add the sour cream, lime juice, Tabasco, and enough chicken broth to thin to a sauce consistency. Season with salt and pepper; add more Tabasco if desired. Thinly slice the chicken, ar-range on plates, and drizzle with the Spicy Avocado Crema.

Spiced Roast Turkey Breast
   The rub from this recipe is also delicious on a boneless roasted turkey breast. Have the butcher cut the meat from the frame of a 2½- to 3-pound turkey breast half for you if you don't want to do it yourself, although it is very simple. Make the spice paste and spread it on the turkey, then roll and tie with cotton string in several places to form an evenly shaped roast. Roast at 400°F for 45 to 60 min-utes, or until the juices run clear or a thermometer reads an internal temperature of 160°F. Slice the roast, arrange on a platter, and serve with the Spicy Avocado Crema as a sauce.

chicken tagine

WLS ½ portion: Calories 164, fat 6.5 gr, carbs 5 gr, protein 16 gr
Serves 4

The turmeric, paprika, and saffron tint the sauce a deep, golden
orange, and the scent of the cumin, ginger, and cinnamon is rich
and sweet in this Moroccan dish. When I serve this dish to my
friends or family, I place a large scoop of couscous in a flat pasta
bowl, topped by chicken, and then ladle on the chunky sauce.
Round out the meal with a simple salad with lemon–olive oil
vinaigrette.

8 large boneless, skinless chicken thighs, about 1½ pounds, cut
   into 2-inch pieces
Kosher salt and freshly ground black pepper
1 tablespoon olive oil
1 large onion, diced
4 garlic cloves, chopped
1 teaspoon ground ginger
1 teaspoon ground cumin
2 teaspoons sweet paprika
1 teaspoon ground turmeric
1 teaspoon ground cinnamon
1 cup chicken broth (see Note, page 127)
½ teaspoon saffron threads
Juice of 2 lemons, about ¼ cup
1 teaspoon cornstarch dissolved in 1 tablespoon water
1 tablespoon lemon zest
½ cup green olive pieces, freshly cut from the pit
   (see Note, page 138)

¼ cup blanched whole almonds
½ cup coarsely chopped flat-leaf parsley

Season the chicken with salt and pepper. Heat the olive oil in a Dutch oven or large nonstick skillet over medium-high heat. Brown the chicken pieces and remove to a plate. Pour off all but 1 tablespoon of the fat and sauté the onion and garlic until translucent, about 4 minutes. Stir in the ginger, cumin, paprika, turmeric, and cinnamon; cook for 1 minute, stirring constantly, and return the chicken to the pot with any accumulated juices. Stir in the broth, saffron, lemon juice, and ½ teaspoon salt; bring to a boil, cover, reduce the heat, and simmer for 35 to 40 minutes, until the chicken is very tender. Stir in the cornstarch mixture to thicken the sauce. Add the lemon zest, olives, almonds, and parsley; simmer for an additional 5 minutes, check the seasonings, and serve.

garlic roasted chicken with black olive tapenade

WLS ½ portion: Calories 151, fat 10 gr, carbs 1.5 gr, protein 14 gr
Serves 4

Black olives add a lot of flavor without high carbohydrates. This olive paste is rich and mellow with a lemon-and-garlic kick. Spread any left over on flatbread crackers. Serve this dish with spinach sautéed in olive oil with garlic, and sliced ripe tomatoes.

3 garlic cloves
Kosher salt

3 tablespoons olive oil

Juice of ½ lemon, about 1 tablespoon

Freshly ground black pepper

8 large boneless, skinless chicken thighs, about 1½ pounds

¾ cup Niçoise olives, pitted (see Note, page 138)

2 anchovy fillets, rinsed

1 tablespoon pine nuts

Preheat the oven to 425°F. Mash 2 garlic cloves with a little salt on a cutting board with the side of a large chef's knife to create a paste. Transfer the garlic paste to a small bowl and blend with 1 tablespoon of the olive oil, 1 teaspoon of the lemon juice, and a few grinds of black pepper. Toss the chicken thighs with the garlic-oil mixture, arrange in a shallow roasting pan, and bake for 30 to 35 minutes, or until the juices run clear. Combine the remaining garlic clove, the remaining 2 teaspoons of lemon juice, the olives, anchovy fillets, and pine nuts in a food processor and pulse until a slightly textured paste forms. Transfer to a small bowl, stir in the remaining 2 tablespoons olive oil, and season with salt and pepper.

Thinly slice the chicken thighs, fan out on each plate, and serve with a few spoonfuls of the black olive tapenade to the side.

milanese chicken sauté

WLS ½ portion: Calories 132, fat 5 gr, carbs 6 gr, protein 14 gr
Serves 4

The inspiration for this recipe was a platter of meltingly tender osso buco, the Milanese veal dish I enjoyed at a New Jersey trattoria just before having my bariatric surgery. The braised shanks had great depth of flavor, but what got me was the sprinkling of gremolata, a mixture of finely chopped garlic, lemon zest, and parsley, that made this simple comfort food memorable.

8 large boneless, skinless chicken thighs, about 1½ pounds, cut
into 2-inch pieces
Kosher salt and freshly ground black pepper
1 tablespoon olive oil
1 large onion, chopped
3 garlic cloves, chopped
1 medium carrot, quartered lengthwise and thinly sliced
½ cup white wine
One 14-ounce can diced tomatoes in juice
1 teaspoon dried thyme
1 bay leaf
Zest of 1 orange, cut with a vegetable peeler, scraped of white
pith, and finely julienned
1 teaspoon cornstarch dissolved in 1 tablespoon water

gremolata

Finely grated zest of 1 lemon
3 tablespoons chopped flat-leaf parsley
1 garlic clove, very finely minced with a pinch of salt

Season the chicken with salt and pepper. Heat the olive oil in a Dutch oven or large nonstick skillet over medium-high heat. Brown the chicken pieces and transfer them to a bowl. Discard all but 1 tablespoon of fat from the pot; add the onion, garlic, and carrot, and cook until softened, about 4 minutes. Add the wine, tomatoes, thyme, bay leaf, orange zest, and the chicken, along with any accumulated juices. Bring to a boil, cover, reduce the heat, and simmer for 35 to 40 minutes, until the chicken is very tender. Stir in the cornstarch mixture to thicken the sauce. Season with salt and pepper. Discard the bay leaf.

Combine the lemon zest, parsley, and garlic for the gremolata, and sprinkle a little over each portion just before serving.

chicken cacciatore

WLS ½ portion: Calories 151, fat 5 gr, carbs 7 gr, protein 15 gr
Serves 4

This was one of my mother's Sunday recipes. You can make this into a stew by cutting boneless, skinless thighs or breasts into 1-inch pieces. This recipe also works perfectly with a whole chicken, cut into serving pieces. Cutting the large breast pieces in half gives you 8 pieces of similar serving size. If you are not a carbohydrate watcher, serve this in a shallow flat bowl on top of a scoop of creamy polenta made with chicken broth and plenty of grated Parmesan. A tossed salad dressed with balsamic vinegar and olive oil completes the meal.

8 large chicken thighs, bone-in, skin removed, about 2 pounds
Kosher salt and freshly ground black pepper
2 teaspoons olive oil
1 medium sweet onion, diced
3 garlic cloves, chopped
4 ounces button or cremini mushrooms, sliced
1 medium green bell pepper, diced
One 14-ounce can crushed tomatoes in puree (see Note, page 148)
1 cup white wine or chicken broth (see Note, page 127)
½ teaspoon dried rosemary, finely chopped
1 teaspoon dried basil

½ teaspoon dried thyme

½ cup pepperoncini (Italian peppers) in vinegar, stemmed,
    seeded, and cut into rings

¼ cup black olive pieces (see Note, page 138)

Season the chicken with salt and pepper. Heat the olive oil in a Dutch
oven or large nonstick skillet over medium-high heat. Brown the
chicken pieces and transfer to a plate. Drain off all but 2 teaspoons
of the oil, and in the oil remaining in the skillet sauté the onion,
garlic, mushrooms, and bell pepper until softened, about 5 minutes.
Add the tomatoes, wine, rosemary, basil, thyme, and the browned
chicken along with any accumulated juices. Cover, reduce the heat,
and simmer for 45 minutes, or until the chicken is tender. Add the
pepperoncini and olives, and simmer for an additional 5 minutes
before serving.

pollo chile verde
(chicken stew with green chiles)

WLS ½ portion: Calories 141, fat 7 gr, carbs 7 gr,
protein 14.5 gr
Serves 4

This Southwestern-style chicken stew was inspired by a dish
I enjoyed at a small trading-post restaurant near the Grand
Canyon. Use any combination of green and yellow peppers
but be aware of the heat if you are straying from the varieties
I suggest. Serve the chile verde in a deep bowl with a drizzle
of lime sour cream. I give my family a large wedge of warm
corn bread and they are very happy people.

8 large boneless, skinless chicken thighs, about 1½ pounds, cut
    into 2-inch pieces

Kosher salt and freshly ground black pepper

All-purpose or Wondra flour for dusting

1 tablespoon olive oil

1 large sweet onion, diced

2 Anaheim green chiles, poblano chiles, or New Mexico green
    chiles, stemmed, seeded, and diced

1 yellow bell pepper, stemmed, seeded, and diced

2 large jalapeño chiles, stemmed, seeded, and diced

4 garlic cloves, chopped

½ teaspoon dried oregano

½ teaspoon ground cumin

1 cup prepared tomatillo salsa or salsa verde (see Note, page 148)

Juice of 1 lime, 1½ to 2 tablespoons

½ cup reduced-fat sour cream

Grated zest of 1 lime

Season the chicken with salt and pepper and dust lightly with flour.
Heat the olive oil in a large nonstick skillet over medium-high heat
and brown the chicken pieces; transfer to a bowl. Pour off all but
2 teaspoons of oil. In the oil remaining in the skillet, sauté the onion,
chiles, bell pepper, jalapeños, and garlic until tender, about 5 minutes. Add the oregano and cumin, and sauté for 1 minute. Stir in the
salsa, lime juice, 1 cup water, and the browned chicken pieces along
with any accumulated juices. Cover the skillet, reduce the heat, and
simmer for 35 to 40 minutes, until the chicken is tender.

Blend the sour cream with the lime zest and juice and drizzle a bit
over each serving.

chicken with
tomato and feta sauce

WLS ½ portion: Calories 160, fat 8 gr, carbs 6 gr, protein 15.5 gr
Serves 4

I love feta cheese! It is tangy, fresh, and creamy with a touch of saltiness. I buy a large chunk at the local bulk foods warehouse store. My friend Constantine goes crazy for the Greek flavors in this dish. Serve with baby spinach sautéed in olive oil with garlic, and orzo pasta.

8 large boneless, skinless chicken thighs, about 1½ pounds
Kosher salt and freshly ground black pepper
All-purpose or Wondra flour for dusting
1 tablespoon olive oil
1 medium onion, finely diced
2 garlic cloves, minced
One 15-ounce can diced tomatoes in puree (see Note, page 148)
½ cup white wine
1 teaspoon dried oregano
¼ teaspoon ground cinnamon
4 ounces feta cheese, drained, rinsed, and crumbled
⅓ cup chopped pitted Kalamata or other brine-cured black olives
    (see Note, page 138)

Season the chicken with salt and pepper and dust lightly with flour. Heat the olive oil in a large nonstick skillet over medium-high heat and cook the chicken until well browned on both sides, about 3 minutes per side; transfer to a serving platter. Sauté the onion and garlic in the oil remaining in the pan until golden. Add the tomatoes, wine, oregano, and cinnamon, and season with black pepper. Return the browned chicken to the skillet with any accumulated juices. Cover, reduce the heat, and simmer for 35 to 40 minutes, until the chicken is tender. Add the feta and olives to the skillet, cover again, and simmer for 10 minutes more, or until the cheese begins to melt into the sauce.

chicken paprikash

WLS ½ portion: Calories 162, fat 7 gr, carbs 9 gr, protein 16 gr
Serves 4

I am always trying new spices and ordering different varieties of the same spice to find new flavors. I order from Penzeys Spices (see Sources, page 303); the online convenience has made it simple for cooks like me to try new varieties of old standbys. Some of my favorite discoveries are different varieties of cinnamon, vanilla, pure ground chili powders, curry powder, and, for this recipe, paprika, all with different flavors and intensities. I order my Hungarian Sweet Paprika from Penzeys, but a good brand, Szeged, is available in most supermarkets. Spices quickly become dusty and flavorless, so be sure your paprika is fresh. For family and friends, serve over egg noodles tossed with butter and poppy seeds, along with some sautéed Brussels sprout halves.

8 large chicken thighs, bone-in with skin removed, about 2 pounds
Kosher salt and freshly ground black pepper
1 teaspoon olive oil
1 large sweet onion, diced
1 garlic clove, chopped
1 red bell pepper, cut into 1-inch dice

1 green bell pepper, cut into 1-inch dice

¼ cup Hungarian sweet paprika

½ teaspoon dried marjoram

½ cup white wine

One 15-ounce can diced tomatoes, drained

½ cup reduced-fat sour cream

2 tablespoons chopped flat-leaf parsley

Season the chicken with salt and pepper. Heat the olive oil in a large nonstick skillet over medium-high heat. Add the chicken and cook until well browned on both sides, about 3 minutes per side; transfer to a platter. Remove and discard all but 1 tablespoon of fat from the pan and sauté the onion, garlic, and peppers until softened and beginning to brown, about 6 minutes. Add 3 tablespoons of the paprika and the marjoram and cook, stirring constantly, for 1 minute. Add the wine, tomatoes, and the chicken pieces with any accumulated juices; bring to a boil, cover, reduce the heat, and simmer for 45 minutes, or until the chicken is very tender. Remove the pan from the heat and transfer the chicken pieces to a platter. Blend the remaining tablespoon of paprika into the sour cream in a small bowl. Stir a large spoonful of the hot sauce into the sour cream and then blend the warmed sour cream mixture back into the sauce in the pot. Stir in the parsley. Add the chicken to the pan and coat with the sauce.

tandoori chicken

WLS ½ portion: Calories 100, fat 3 gr, carbs 3 gr, protein 15 gr
Serves 4

The yogurt in the marinade tenderizes the chicken and provides a creamy sauce to moisten the already very juicy meat. I serve this dish to my family with steamed jasmine rice and roasted asparagus spears. This recipe requires advance preparation.

8 large chicken thighs, bone-in with skin removed, about 2 pounds

½-inch piece fresh ginger, peeled and chopped

½ small onion, chopped

2 garlic cloves, chopped

½ cup low-fat yogurt

1 tablespoon Hungarian sweet paprika

1 teaspoon garam masala (see Note, page 160)

1 teaspoon ground cumin

1 teaspoon ground coriander

¼ teaspoon cayenne

½ teaspoon kosher salt

1 tablespoon lemon juice (about ½ lemon)

Vegetable oil cooking spray

½ cup low-sodium chicken broth

Make deep cuts 1 inch apart on the surface of the chicken pieces, slicing almost to the bone. Puree the ginger, onion, and garlic with the yogurt in a food processor or blender and blend in the paprika, garam masala, cumin, coriander, cayenne, salt, and lemon juice, to make a smooth paste. Pour the mixture over the chicken pieces in a ceramic or plastic bowl, turning to coat; cover and refrigerate for 2 to 8 hours.

Preheat the oven to 450°F. Place the chicken pieces, coated with the thick marinade, in a lightly oiled baking pan and roast for 35 minutes, or until the juices run clear. Transfer the chicken to a platter and add the chicken broth to the hot pan, whisking to slightly emulsify the juices into a sauce and scraping up any browned bits. Pour some of the sauce over the chicken.

sesame roasted chicken

WLS ½ portion: Calories 151, fat 10 gr, carbs <1 gr,
protein 14 gr
Serves 4

The sesame dressing used to marinate the chicken thighs is one
of the most versatile sauces in this book. (This recipe makes
about ¾ cup.) Keep a container of it in your refrigerator. For a
quick lunch, I blend a tablespoon of the sesame dressing with one
teaspoon of mayonnaise and mix it into a pouch of albacore tuna
or chopped rotisserie chicken. I toss in a few handfuls of baby
greens with a little of this dressing. Marinate game hens in some
of the dressing before grilling, or drizzle it over roasted, sliced
chicken. Use it on grilled or broiled seafood, too. Quickly sauté
a pound of peeled and cleaned shrimp and add enough of the
sesame marinade to coat for a simple salad.

Makes a great meal when served with Yukon gold mashed
potatoes and baby greens dressed with some of the remaining
marinade. This recipe requires advance preparation.

sesame marinade/dressing

3 tablespoons toasted sesame oil

3 tablespoons peanut oil

2 tablespoons soy sauce

3 tablespoons rice vinegar

1 tablespoon Splenda Granular

2 teaspoons whole sesame seeds

Freshly ground black pepper
8 large chicken thighs, about 2 pounds

In a small bowl, whisk together the sesame and peanut oils, soy sauce, vinegar, Splenda, sesame seeds, and pepper to taste until emulsified. Pour ½ cup of the marinade over the chicken thighs in a shallow bowl or plastic bag; set the rest of the marinade aside. Cover and refrigerate the chicken for 2 to 8 hours.

Preheat the oven to 425°F. Arrange the marinated chicken pieces in a small shallow pan skin side up, and roast for 30 to 35 minutes, until the juices run clear when pierced with the tip of a knife. Drizzle a little of the reserved marinade over the chicken just before serving.

asian meatballs
with peanut sauce

WLS ½ portion (3 meatballs): Calories 115, fat 6 gr, carbs 3.5 gr, protein 10 gr
Makes 24 meatballs; serves 4

This recipe combines my favorite flavors, sesame and ginger, with the unexpected mellowness of peanut butter flavoring the sauce. I serve this dish with an Asian coleslaw: dress a bag of preshredded cabbage with 2 tablespoons each of rice vinegar and peanut oil and 1 teaspoon sesame oil, and sprinkle with sesame seeds.

2 tablespoons peanut butter (any variety in your pantry is fine)
1 tablespoon soy sauce
2 teaspoons sesame oil (I use hot pepper sesame oil)
½ cup chicken broth or water

1 pound ground chicken or turkey breast
½ cup finely chopped green onions (scallions)
1 teaspoon garlic chile paste (available in the Asian section)
2 teaspoons grated peeled ginger
1 tablespoon soy sauce
¼ cup plain bread crumbs
Nonstick vegetable oil spray

Blend the peanut butter, soy sauce, sesame oil, and broth in a small bowl and set aside.

Combine the ground chicken with the green onions, chile paste, ginger, soy sauce, and bread crumbs until well combined. Divide the chicken mixture into 1-tablespoon portions, and roll into balls. Spray a nonstick skillet with cooking spray and sauté the meatballs over medium-high heat until golden brown on both sides and cooked through, 3 to 4 minutes. Pour the sauce into the pan, lower the heat, and gently cook until bubbling, adding water to bring the sauce to the desired consistency. Roll the meatballs in the sauce to coat them thoroughly.

buffalo simmered chicken

WLS ½ portion (1 thigh): Calories 82, fat 3 gr, carbs 2 gr, protein 16 gr
Serves 4

I love the flavors of Buffalo wings, but they are too greasy and have too much skin for me to eat. So I translated the ingredients into simmered tender chunks of chicken, and added a homemade blue-cheese dressing to take it over the top. This dish is fantastic using tilapia fillets. Lightly dust the fish fillets with Wondra or all-purpose flour and sauté them in a tablespoon of olive oil in a nonstick skillet before dousing them in wing sauce. Don't forget the homemade blue-cheese dressing.

2 pounds boneless skinless chicken thighs, about 8 thighs
Nonstick vegetable oil spray
1 cup chicken broth (see Note, page 127)
½ cup Frank's Red Hot Buffalo Wing sauce (not the regular hot sauce)
Kosher salt and freshly ground black pepper
Classic Blue Cheese Dip (recipe follows)

Cut the thighs in half and brown in a nonstick skillet coated in vegetable spray. Add the broth and half of the wing sauce. Cover and simmer until the chicken is very tender and the sauce is thickened, 35 to 40 minutes. Add the remaining wing sauce and season with salt and pepper. Serve drizzled with homemade Classic Blue Cheese Dip.

classic blue cheese dip

WLS portion (1 tablespoon): Calories 79, fat 3 gr, carbs 1 gr, protein 1 gr
Makes about 1 cup

Once you make this homemade dressing and see how easy it is, you will never be able to eat bottled blue-cheese dressing again.

4 ounces blue cheese, crumbled
3 tablespoons milk
½ cup reduced-fat or light mayonnaise
2 tablespoons white vinegar

1 teaspoon Dijon mustard
⅛ teaspoon kosher salt
⅛ teaspoon freshly ground black pepper

Using a fork, mash the blue cheese with the milk in a small bowl until creamy. Whisk in the mayonnaise, vinegar, mustard, salt, and pepper. Cover and refrigerate.

parmesan-crusted
chicken tenders

WLS ½ serving (two 3-ounce pieces): Calories 208, fat 8 gr, carbs 5 gr, protein 22 gr
Serves 2

After a busy day at work, I discovered that I had forgotten to transfer a package of chicken from the freezer to the refrigerator that morning. Not having anything else to prepare, I placed the frozen chicken pieces in a bowl of water to thaw while I prepared the other ingredients for our supper. Not only did the water quickly thaw the chicken, but it also infused extra moisture into the meat! Now I plan a brief soak for my chicken tenders for extra-moist and juicy meat.

10 ounces chicken tenders, 7 to 8 pieces
2 tablespoons kosher salt
¼ cup mayonnaise
¼ cup grated Parmesan cheese
½ cup Italian-flavored bread crumbs or Japanese panko
**   bread crumbs**

Preheat the oven to 425°F. In a large bowl, dissolve the salt in a small amount of hot water, then fill the bowl two-thirds full with cold water. Place the chicken tenders in the water and soak for 10 to 15 minutes. Remove the tenders from the brining solution, drain well, and pat dry with paper towels.

Combine the mayonnaise and cheese in a small bowl. Add the chicken pieces to the bowl and toss to coat each tender with the mayonnaise mixture. Lightly roll in the bread crumbs and place on a foil-lined baking sheet. Bake for 10 to 12 minutes, until almost cooked through; turn on the broiler and continue to cook until golden brown, 1 to 2 minutes.

pineapple chicken

WLS portion (4 ounces): Calories 185, fat 8 gr, carbs 5 gr, protein 22 gr
Serves 4

This marinade was inspired by the roasted salmon dish we enjoyed in Las Vegas at the MGM Grand's Shibuya Japanese sushi restaurant. The salmon had not arrived yet at the fish market, so I made the dish with chicken and it was excellent. Make an extra portion of either chicken or salmon to use in a wrap or salad for the next day's lunch. This is especially delicious with spinach sautéed in garlic and sesame oil.

One 8-ounce can Libby's Splenda-sweetened crushed pineapple
¼ cup soy sauce
½ teaspoon sesame oil
½ teaspoon minced garlic

½ teaspoon grated peeled ginger
1 whole chicken, cut up, or 8 chicken thighs, skin removed

Blend together the pineapple with juice, soy sauce, sesame oil, garlic, and ginger in a medium bowl. Add the chicken pieces to the marinade and turn to coat. Marinate for 2 to 4 hours or overnight in the refrigerator.

Preheat the oven to 400°F. Arrange the chicken pieces in a shallow roasting pan; spoon on the remaining marinade. Roast for 50 to 60 minutes, basting occasionally with pan juices, until the chicken pieces are tender and cooked through.

orange teriyaki game hens

WLS ½ portion: Calories 186, fat 5 gr, carbs 9 gr, protein 25 gr
Serves 4

Game hens are very moist and juicy, an ideal protein food for post-surgery diners. These birds are particularly succulent after an overnight soak in this Asian-flavored marinade. For hearty eaters, double the marinade and serve a whole hen to each person. This recipe requires advance preparation.

For guests, pair the hens with wasabi mashed potatoes and sautéed snow peas. To make the wasabi potatoes, blend boiled and riced Yukon gold potatoes with butter, milk, salt and pepper to taste, sliced green onions (scallions), and a tablespoon of prepared wasabi paste.

¾ cup orange juice
3 tablespoons soy sauce
¼ cup Nature's Hollow Apricot Preserves

2 tablespoons toasted sesame oil
2 garlic cloves, minced
1 tablespoon grated peeled ginger
Two 20- to 24-ounce Cornish game hens, split in half

Blend together the orange juice, soy sauce, preserves, sesame oil, garlic, and ginger and pour over the hens in a shallow bowl or plastic bag. Cover and refrigerate for 2 to 24 hours, preferably overnight.

Preheat the oven to 400°F. Drain the hens, reserving the marinade; arrange in a baking dish skin side up and roast for 35 to 40 minutes, until the juices run clear and the skin is golden. Reduce the reserved marinade in a small saucepan over medium-high heat until a thick glaze forms. Drizzle a little glaze over the roasted hens just before serving.

grandma's lemon game hens

WLS ½ portion: Calories 269, fat 16 gr, carbs 1.5 gr, protein 24 gr
Serves 4

My grandma Helen makes the most delicious, juicy roasted lemon- and oregano-flavored hens you have ever tasted. She doesn't measure anything, of course, so I had to watch her half a dozen times to get the right proportions. For those not watching their carbohydrate intake, mashed potatoes taste wonderful mixed with some of the lemon sauce. Add a tossed salad dressed with balsamic vinegar and olive oil.

½ cup lemon juice (about 4 lemons)
¼ cup olive oil

2 teaspoons balsamic vinegar
2 garlic cloves, minced
1 teaspoon dried oregano
Kosher salt and freshly ground black pepper
Two 20- to 24-ounce Cornish game hens, split in half
¼ cup chopped flat-leaf parsley

Preheat the oven to 425°F. In a large bowl, whisk together the lemon juice, olive oil, vinegar, garlic, and oregano, and season with salt and pepper. Loosen the skin on the hens but do not remove. Toss the hens with the lemon dressing; arrange skin side up in a shallow roasting pan. Pour all of the dressing from the bowl over the hens. Roast for 30 to 35 minutes, basting after 15 minutes, until the juices run clear and the skin is nicely browned. Transfer the hens to a serving platter and pour the lemon sauce and juices into a small saucepan. Bring the sauce to a boil and reduce until slightly thickened. Stir in the parsley, spoon a little sauce over the game hens, and serve the rest in a small bowl for pouring at the table.

turkey tenderloins with creamy roasted garlic vegetable sauté

WLS portion (3½ ounces): Calories 225, fat 8 gr, carbs 5 gr, protein 32 gr
Serves 4

What was I thinking when I ordered an entire case of garlic from an Oregon farm? For a week, I experimented with roasted garlic until I came up with the perfect recipe. My husband loves to dig into a bowl of this dip with my homemade baked spiced pita chips. I cut pita rounds into wedges, lightly brush the pieces with olive oil, sprinkle them with chipotle chile powder and salt, and bake them at 350°F until golden brown and crisp. Combined with sautéed zucchini and red peppers, the resulting creamy vegetable salsa is equally good on a piece of roasted mahimahi.

1 whole large garlic bulb

2 turkey tenderloins, about 1½ pounds

2 teaspoons olive oil, plus extra to coat the tenderloins

Kosher salt and freshly ground black pepper

4 ounces (¼ pound) reduced-fat cream cheese

¼ cup reduced-fat sour cream

2 tablespoons chopped roasted red peppers

2 green onions (scallions), thinly sliced, including green tops

¼ teaspoon dried thyme

¼ teaspoon dried basil

½ teaspoon Worcestershire sauce

3 medium zucchini, cut lengthwise into planks, then diced

1 small red bell pepper, cut into ½-inch dice

Preheat the oven to 400°F. Tightly wrap the entire garlic bulb in foil and roast for 1 hour. Remove the garlic from the oven and loosen the foil. When the bulb is cool enough to handle, squeeze the roasted garlic from each clove into a small bowl and set aside.

Rub the turkey tenderloins with olive oil, season with salt and pepper, and roast in a shallow baking pan at 400°F for 30 to 45 minutes, until the juices run clear and the meat reaches an internal temperature of 160°F on an instant-read thermometer.

Puree the roasted garlic, cream cheese, sour cream, roasted peppers, green onions, thyme, basil, and Worcestershire in a blender or food processor until creamy; add salt and pepper to taste. Heat 2 teaspoons olive oil in a nonstick skillet over medium-high heat and sauté the zucchini and bell pepper until very tender and starting to brown, 5 to 6 minutes; remove from the heat, add the creamy roasted garlic mixture, and fold it into the vegetables as it melts. Thinly slice the roasted tenderloins and spoon on some of the creamy roasted garlic vegetable sauté.

rolled boneless turkey breast with apples and sage

WLS portion (4 ounces): Calories 185, fat 4 gr, carbs 5 gr, protein 33 gr
Serves 4

When I make a special holiday meal for just the two of us I don't need a whole turkey—or a whole lot of food, for that matter. My grocery store sells turkey parts, so I can buy a turkey breast half that weighs about 2½ to 3 pounds, perfect for dinner plus leftovers. Once again, don't overcook your turkey. A turkey breast should roast until a meat thermometer reads 160°F so it stays moist inside.

One 2½- to 3-pound boneless turkey breast half, butterflied
    (either have it boned or do it yourself)
Olive oil
Bell's Seasoning, or your favorite prepared poultry blend
Garlic powder
Kosher salt and freshly ground black pepper
1 Granny Smith apple, peeled, cored, and very thinly sliced
½ cup chicken broth

If you are boning your own turkey breast half, it is easier to place the meat skin side down on the cutting board and, using the tip of a sharp knife, cut and lift the bones away from the meat.

Preheat the oven to 325°F.

With the skin side down, lightly coat the meat with olive oil, then sprinkle generously with Bell's Seasoning, garlic powder, salt, and pepper. Tuck a few of the apple slices down the center of the roast, and fold up both sides, encasing the apple and seasonings in the center of the roast. Tie with cotton kitchen string in several places. Place seam side down in a shallow roasting pan. Coat the skin with olive oil and season with salt and pepper. Arrange the remaining apple slices around the roast in the pan. Roast until a meat thermometer inserted into the center of the meat reads 160°F, about 1 hour. Mash the apple slices into the pan juices using a fork, then add ½ cup of chicken broth for a moist and delicious sauce for the sliced turkey.

turkey tenderloin with apple chipotle chutney

WLS portion (3 ounces turkey, ¼ cup chutney): Calories 210, fat 7 gr, carbs 7 gr, protein 25 gr
Serves 4; makes 2 cups chutney

I was sent a gift bottle of apple chipotle cooking sauce, but upon reading the label I discovered it contained far too much sugar for me to even consider a taste. Everyone who picked up the bottle and read *apple and chipotle* made some sort of noise of approval, then was sad to see the amount of sugar, knowing I couldn't eat it. I also thought that apples and chipotle sounded like a tasty combination and set out to create a dish.

The chutney-style apple chipotle condiment would also be perfect served as an accompaniment to a Thanksgiving turkey, grilled tenderized chicken cutlets, a grilled turkey burger, or even tender lamb chops.

Two turkey tenderloins, about 2½ to 3 pounds total
2 tablespoons olive oil
Kosher salt and freshly ground black pepper
3 large apples, peeled and diced (golden Delicious and Granny
**   Smith have both produced superb results)**
1 medium onion, diced
1 to 2 teaspoons ground chipotle chile (or 1 to 2 mashed canned
**   chipotle in adobo sauce; see Sources, page 303)**
½ to 1 cup chicken broth

Preheat the oven to 400°F. Match up the turkey tenderloins by placing the thick end of one with the smaller end of the other and tying them with cotton kitchen string in intervals to make one evenly shaped roast (see Note). Alternatively, you can fold under the thinner third of each tenderloin, creating two smaller but more evenly shaped pieces for cooking. Brush with olive oil, sprinkle with salt and pepper, and set aside.

Heat the remaining oil in a nonstick skillet over medium-high heat and sauté the apples and onions until golden, 5 to 6 minutes. Stir in the chipotle and ½ cup of the broth. Cover the skillet, reduce the heat, and simmer until the mixture is very soft and has thickened, 15 to 20 minutes. Add up to ½ cup more broth to bring to the desired consistency.

Roast the prepared turkey tenderloins to 160°F on an instant-read meat thermometer inserted into the thickest portion of the tenderloin. Remove from the oven, cover, and allow the meat to rest before carving into thin slices. Serve a few slices with the apple chutney.

Note: When I am buying meat or poultry that I think I will need to tie or truss, I ring the bell at the supermarket meat counter and ask for a length of cotton kitchen string. If you have never tied turkey tenderloins, or boned a turkey breast, ask the butcher to do it for you; they are usually happy to oblige. When you get home, you can inspect the results so next time you'll know what to do on your own. Don't be shy to ask for help.

turkey burgers
with muffuletta salad

WLS ½ portion: Calories 112.5, fat 8 gr, carbs 1 gr, protein 10.5 gr
Serves 4

I used to make big, round sourdough sandwiches with Italian cold cuts and a thick layer of this olive salad. In New Orleans, this sandwich is called a muffuletta. Although my big sandwich days are in the past, I wanted to use the same flavors of the salad as a condiment to moisten a burger. Adding shredded cheese keeps the burger from getting too solid and dry. My family enjoys their turkey burgers piled with the salad on a chewy sourdough roll, with hand-cut potato chips, while I eat mine without the bread with a little of the salad spooned over it. Also try this salad with broiled or grilled chicken, or roasted or sautéed fish. Lightly dust flounder fillets with seasoned Italian bread crumbs, sauté in olive oil, and top with the muffuletta salad.

muffuletta salad

½ cup finely diced artichoke hearts, canned or frozen (thawed)
¼ cup finely diced roasted red or yellow peppers

¼ cup pitted and chopped Sicilian green olives (see Note, page 138)

¼ cup pitted and chopped oil-cured black olives

1 garlic clove, minced

¼ cup chopped flat-leaf parsley

2 tablespoons olive oil

2 teaspoons balsamic vinegar

Juice of ½ lemon, about 1 tablespoon

Kosher salt and freshly ground black pepper

turkey burgers

1 pound lean ground turkey

1 egg, lightly beaten

½ cup packaged Italian-style bread crumbs

½ cup shredded Cheddar cheese

In a large bowl, combine the artichokes, peppers, olives, garlic, parsley, olive oil, vinegar, and lemon juice; season with salt and pepper, and set aside.

Preheat the grill or broiler. Mix the turkey, egg, bread crumbs, and cheese in a large bowl, using your hands to combine gently. Shape into four ½-inch-thick patties. Grill or broil the patties until cooked through but still moist, 3 to 4 minutes per side. Serve with a little of the marinated salad piled on top of each burger.

turkey mushroom meat loaf

WLS ½ portion: Calories 143, fat 7 gr, carbs 4 gr, protein 15 gr
Serves 4

This meat loaf is very moist, tender, and easy to eat. A classic served with mashed Yukon gold potatoes and green beans for the family. Early after my surgery, I would mash together a small piece of the meat loaf with a spoonful of the pan gravy and a few green beans; not a very attractive mixture, but it tasted great and had the perfect texture.

2 teaspoons olive oil
1 medium onion, finely diced
2 garlic cloves, minced
8 ounces cremini, portobello, or button mushrooms, finely diced
1 slice firm white or wheat bread
1¼ pounds lean ground turkey
¼ cup coarsely chopped flat-leaf parsley
1 large egg
½ teaspoon kosher salt
¼ teaspoon freshly ground black pepper
½ teaspoon dried thyme

Preheat the oven to 350°F. Heat the olive oil in a nonstick skillet over medium-high heat and sauté the onion and garlic until lightly browned, about 4 minutes. Add the mushrooms and cook, stirring occasionally, about 4 minutes, until the released liquid has been reduced to a glaze. Crumble the bread into a small bowl, moisten with ½ cup water, and mash with a fork into a coarse paste. In a large bowl, gently combine the ground turkey, bread, sautéed vegetables, parsley, egg, salt, pepper, and thyme. Spoon into a 9 × 5 × 3–inch loaf pan, smooth the top, and bake for 45 to 50 minutes, until the juices run clear and the internal temperature reaches 160°F, measured at the center with an instant-read thermometer.

italian meatballs

WLS ½ portion (2 meatballs): Calories 110, fat 8 gr, carbs 10 gr, protein 17 gr
Serves 6

When my father retired and moved to Florida, I revived our family tradition of the Sunday spaghetti dinner. Since my bariatric surgery, I no longer enjoy pasta because of the carbohydrates, and the texture and consistency do not agree with me. I substituted ground turkey for the first few months post-op as it is easier to digest, but now I am back to using equal amounts of lean ground beef and pork. My family enjoys their sauce and meatballs on a plate of perfectly cooked spaghetti or ziti, but I am perfectly satisfied with one or two small meatballs napped with a little sauce and topped with some freshly grated Parmesan. I also serve a crusty Italian loaf and a salad of baby greens, tomatoes, olives, and artichoke hearts, tossed with olive oil and balsamic vinegar.

meatballs

1¼ pounds ground lean turkey

1 large egg, lightly beaten

2 tablespoons freshly grated Parmesan

½ teaspoon dried thyme

½ teaspoon kosher salt

½ teaspoon freshly ground black pepper

2 garlic cloves, minced

½ cup coarsely chopped flat-leaf parsley

½ cup packaged Italian-style bread crumbs mixed with ½ cup water

1 tablespoon olive oil

sauce for italian meatballs and spaghetti

1 tablespoon olive oil

1 medium onion, diced

3 garlic cloves, chopped

One 28-ounce can crushed tomatoes

One 28-ounce can tomato puree

One 6-ounce can tomato paste

1 tablespoon dried basil

½ teaspoon dried thyme

½ teaspoon dried oregano

¼ teaspoon crushed red pepper flakes

Kosher salt and freshly ground black pepper

Combine the turkey with the egg, cheese, thyme, salt, pepper, garlic, parsley, and bread crumbs in a large bowl until very well blended. Roll the mixture into about 24 balls, 1½ inches in diameter. Heat 1 tablespoon of olive oil in a nonstick skillet over medium-high heat and brown the meatballs on all sides. Transfer to a bowl and set aside.

Heat 1 tablespoon of olive oil over medium-high heat in a Dutch oven or deep saucepan. Sauté the onion until softened, about 4 minutes; add the garlic and sauté for an additional 2 minutes, stirring constantly. Add the crushed tomatoes, tomato puree, tomato paste, basil, thyme, oregano, and red pepper flakes. Season with salt and pepper. Stir in 1 cup water, bring to a boil, reduce the heat to low, and simmer for 45 minutes, stirring occasionally. Add the meatballs, along with any accumulated juices from the bowl, cover, and simmer for an additional 45 minutes. Ladle the sauce over the pasta and serve with the meatballs.

desserts

So many people think that their pre-op eating frenzy of chocolate cake and Häagen-Dazs will be the last desserts of their life. Our relationship with cake and ice cream is forever changed by our surgery, but we can have an occasional dessert as long as we watch our sugar intake. Since my surgery, I no longer live to eat, and my tastes truly have changed. Sweets taste much sweeter, and I don't crave Entenmanns's Ultimate Crumb Cake anymore . . . at least, not the entire cake. I still love food and flavors, but I am satisfied with a small amount. I savor each bite instead of thinking about another plateful. I don't make dessert every night; I don't even make it twice a week. I make dessert occasionally when we have friends over for dinner, or when my girlfriends come and we sit on my patio and talk all afternoon, or when I have prepared a special dinner, or when I just want to treat my husband and myself. Incredible sugar-free desserts for special occasions can still be a part of our lives after our surgery. When I dine in a fine restaurant I will have one small bite of my husband's decadent dessert, but at home I prefer to make something sugar-free.

I don't want to cross the line into "dumping" territory, so I stay well under 10 grams of sugar in one serving of any food; usually I am in the 5-grams-or-fewer zone to be safe. At home I can prepare desserts that have essentially 0 grams of sugar. It is an added chal-

lenge to keep desserts not only sugar-free but also low in carbohydrates. Every recipe in this cookbook has fewer than 15 grams
of carbohydrates—most have fewer than 10 grams per serving—and
that holds true for the desserts as well. I baked the blueberry cheesecake to take to a friend's home for her Christmas sweets table and it
was the hit of the holiday! No one could believe that my light and
creamy dessert was sugar-free and low-fat.

I have two sweeteners of choice depending on the type of recipe.
Splenda is an excellent sugar substitute. It tastes and measures like
sugar, yet doesn't have the carbohydrates or the calories. The granulated version that is packaged in boxes and bags works perfectly in
recipes in which the sugar doesn't provide the framework for the
dessert, such as custards, creams, and fruit sauces. I use it in sweetened recipes that are creamy or wet; but it is not my first choice for
baking.

Do not accidentally use Splenda Sugar Blend for Baking or
Splenda Brown Sugar Blend products thinking that they are sugar-
free and acceptable for our use. Regular Splenda doesn't produce a
good result when substituted for sugar in cake or cookie recipes, so
the manufacturer created these two products blending Splenda with
granulated or brown sugar as reduced-sugar versions that work when
baking. I think these products are a terrible idea, because too many
people do not realize that these blends, labeled with the Splenda
name, contain real sugar. The nutritional statistics on the package do
not clarify the nature of this product; the label says that one serving
contains just 2 grams of sugar, but people do not normally notice that
the serving size is ½ *teaspoon*. I get numerous e-mails from people
who find these blends and are excited to tell me about them. They
have no idea that they are using real sugar. I am certain that this is
problematic for diabetics as well. Always read labels carefully, read
ingredient lists, and check serving sizes.

Truvia Baking Blend is the sugar replacer that I use for baking. It is a natural sugar-free sweetener that uses stevia leaf. This product has the same bulk and weight as sugar and works perfectly in baking. It creams with the butter and eggs as sugar does; it provides bulk and lift when the flour is incorporated into the mixture. Truvia Baking Blend contains erythritol and too large a portion can create a laxative effect in those people who are sensitive to sugar alcohols.

The nutritional analysis for each dessert is for a full portion based on the serving size.

belgian chocolate cheesecake

Full portion: Calories 173, fat 4.3 gr, carbs 7 gr, protein 6 gr
Serves 12

A perfect dessert. The chocolate flavor of the filling is intense; the chocolate cookie crust gives it an added boost of chocolate crunch; and it's sugar free.

1 cup Joseph's Sugar-Free Chocolate Walnut cookies (bite-size) (see Note, page 241)
1 tablespoon salted butter, melted
1 pound reduced-fat cream cheese
1 cup Splenda Granular
¼ cup reduced-fat sour cream
2 large eggs
1 large egg yolk
3 ounces sugar-free dark chocolate (Valor or Guylian are excellent, see Note, page 241), broken into pieces and microwaved on medium for 60 seconds, or until just melted

1 teaspoon vanilla extract
Raspberry Sauce (recipe follows)

Preheat the oven to 325°F. Place the cookies in a food processor and pulse with the butter until you have moist, fine crumbs. Press evenly into an 8-inch springform pan or pie plate and bake for 10 to 12 minutes, until the crust just starts to color. Cool on a rack while preparing the filling. (Leave the oven on at 325°F.)

Beat the cream cheese until smooth with an electric mixer; add the Splenda Granular, sour cream, eggs, egg yolk, melted chocolate, and vanilla, in order, beating thoroughly after each addition. Scrape down the bowl and blend again until smooth. Pour into the crust and bake for 30 minutes, or until the center is barely set. Transfer to a cooling rack and run the thin blade of a knife around the edges of the cheesecake to loosen it from the springform pan (to prevent the cake from cracking). Cool to room temperature; chill at least 2 hours before serving. Serve small wedges with Splenda-sweetened raspberry sauce.

raspberry sauce

10 ounces frozen raspberries (Cascadian Farm 100% Organic
      Frozen Red Raspberries are so good and convenient that I
      rarely use fresh berries)
¼ cup Splenda Granular, plus more to taste
Pinch of table salt
1 teaspoon fresh lime juice

In a medium saucepan, bring the berries, 2 tablespoons water, the Splenda, and salt to a simmer over medium heat, stirring occasionally until the berries have softened and released their juice, about 2 minutes. Transfer the berry mixture to a food processor or blender and puree until smooth. Strain through a fine-mesh strainer into a small bowl, pressing the puree through the strainer with a rubber spatula. Stir in the lime juice, and add additional Splenda if desired. Cover and chill.

Note: Joseph's makes an excellent line of sugar-free cookies that are widely available in grocery stores. They are all natural and quite tasty. I keep several varieties on hand for sugar-free snacking and as a dessert ingredient. For a quick cream pie, I prepare a simple crumb crust using the cookies and fill it with cooked sugar-free pudding livened up with a dash of vanilla extract. A small chilled wedge served with a squirt of Reddi-wip is a great treat. Chocolate cream and banana cream pie are childhood comfort foods and my version is sugar free. Joseph's sugar-free cookies are also available at www.BariatricEating.com.

The creaminess and flavor of imported chocolate valor is remarkable, and it is becoming more readily available at grocery, rather than just specialty, stores. If you can't find it locally, it can be ordered online at BariatricEating.com.

blueberry cheesecake

Full portion: Calories 163, fat 12 gr, carbs 8 gr, protein 6 gr
Serves 12

Cheesecake is my ultimate holiday and special-occasion dessert. You can either spread the blueberry compote on top of the cake for a beautiful whole cake presentation, or you can serve the cake in small wedges on dessert plates and spoon some of the topping over the slice.

1 cup Joseph's Sugar-Free Lemon cookies (see Note, above)
1 tablespoon salted butter, melted
1 pound reduced-fat cream cheese

1 cup Splenda Granular

1 tablespoon vanilla extract

1 teaspoon fresh lemon juice

½ cup reduced-fat sour cream

2 large eggs

1 large egg yolk

blueberry topping

1 cup fresh blueberries or unthawed frozen blueberries

2 tablespoons fresh orange juice

1 teaspoon cornstarch

2 tablespoons Splenda Granular

¼ teaspoon freshly grated orange zest

Preheat the oven to 325°F. Place the cookies in a food processor and pulse with the butter until you have moist, fine crumbs. Press evenly into an 8-inch springform pan or pie plate and bake for 10 to 12 minutes, until the crust just starts to color. Cool on a rack while preparing the filling. (Leave the oven on at 325°F.)

Beat the cream cheese with an electric mixer until smooth; add the Splenda, vanilla, lemon juice, sour cream, eggs, and egg yolk, in order, beating thoroughly after each addition. Scrape down the bowl and blend again until smooth. Pour into the crust and bake for 30 minutes, or until the center is barely set. Transfer to a rack to cool to room temperature.

Simmer the blueberries with 1 tablespoon of the orange juice in a small saucepan over medium-high heat. In a separate bowl, blend the cornstarch with the remaining tablespoon of orange juice and add to the blueberries; stir constantly until the mixture comes to a boil and becomes glossy and thick. Remove from the heat and stir in the Splenda and orange zest. Let cool slightly while the cheesecake comes to room temperature. Spread the blueberry sauce just to the edges of the cake and refrigerate at least 2 hours before cutting and serving.

chocolate génoise

Full portion: Calories 107, fat 7 gr, carbs 7.5 gr, protein 5.2 gr
Serves 10

A génoise is a moist cake with a tender crumb. The Dutch-processed cocoa gives it a deep, dark chocolate flavor. I serve it with just a dusting of confectioners' sugar. Take this basic chocolate layer over the top by making it into a sugar-free Black Forest Torte. Spoon a little sugar-free cherry pie filling over a wedge of chocolate génoise, dust the edge with confectioners' sugar, and top with Splenda-sweetened whipped cream.

The secret to making this cake is in the beating of the eggs. I use a medium glass bowl and set it over a saucepan of barely simmering water while I beat the eggs with my handheld electric mixer. The first time you make this recipe you will be amazed that you can whip eggs into a bowl of whipped cream–like silky foam. Be patient, as it does take 12 to 15 minutes. This cake must be refrigerated after the first 24 hours.

Vegetable oil cooking spray
½ cup all-purpose flour
½ cup Dutch-processed unsweetened cocoa (Droste is an excellent brand)
6 large eggs, at room temperature
1 cup Splenda Granular

1 teaspoon vanilla extract

2 tablespoons salted butter, melted

Preheat the oven to 350°F. Spray the bottom and sides of a 9-inch round cake pan with cooking spray, line the bottom with a round of wax paper, and spray again.

Sift the flour and cocoa together into a large bowl using a fine-mesh strainer and set aside.

Combine the eggs and Splenda in a glass bowl, beating with an electric mixer on high until doubled in volume, about 5 minutes. Set the bowl over a pan of simmering water to slightly warm the egg mixture, and continue beating for an additional 5 to 7 minutes, until the mixture is the consistency of softly whipped cream. Beat in the vanilla.

Lightly fold the flour and cocoa into the eggs, about one third at a time, using a large rubber scraper and cutting through the batter, being careful not to deflate the mixture too much. Fold in the butter until just incorporated and pour into the prepared pan.

Bake for 15 minutes, or until a toothpick inserted in the center comes out clean. Cool for 10 minutes, turn out onto a cake rack, and carefully peel off the paper.

lemon-almond sponge cake

Full portion: Calories 129, fat 9 gr, carbs 7 gr, protein 6 gr
Serves 10

I didn't have a low-carbohydrate, sugar-free sponge cake to use as a base for my husband's beloved strawberry shortcake. So whenever I would indulge Ty, I ate just a few berries with a dab of Splenda-sweetened whipped cream. While I was experimenting with almond flour, using the principles for making a génoise, I came up with this moist, lemony cake. In addition to being a delicious cake to enjoy with a cup of tea, this is the perfect base for my sugar-free strawberry shortcake. I slice a quart of ripe berries and puree ½ cup of the berries with ¼ cup of Nature's Hollow Strawberry Preserves in a food processor, and then fold the puree back into the remaining berries. Spoon this compote on top of a thin wedge of the lemon-almond sponge cake and top with a generous dollop of Splenda-sweetened whipped cream.

You must use an electric mixer to whip the eggs. This cake can be made in advance and freezes beautifully as well. It must be refrigerated after the first 24 hours.

Vegetable oil cooking spray
3 large eggs, at room temperature
¾ cup Splenda Granular
1 teaspoon vanilla extract
1 teaspoon lemon extract
3 large egg whites, at room temperature
¼ teaspoon cream of tartar
¾ cup almond flour (see Note)
½ cup all-purpose flour
1½ tablespoons salted butter, melted

Preheat the oven to 375°F. Lightly spray the bottom and sides of a 9-inch cake pan with cooking spray, line the bottom of the pan with a round of wax paper, and spray again.

Combine the whole eggs with ½ cup of the Splenda in a medium bowl. Beat using an electric mixer until the mixture is the consistency of softly whipped cream and is triple in volume, about 12 minutes. Beat in the vanilla and lemon extracts. Using clean beaters, beat the egg whites with the cream of tartar in a medium bowl until soft peaks form. Gradually add the remaining ¼ cup Splenda and continue beating until stiff but not dry. Fold the whites into the egg mixture.

In a small bowl, blend the almond flour with the all-purpose flour and gently fold into the egg mixture until incorporated. Fold in the melted butter. Pour the batter into the prepared pan and smooth the top. Bake for 18 to 20 minutes, until a toothpick inserted into the center of the cake comes out clean. Cool for 10 minutes, then turn the cake out onto a rack and remove the wax paper.

Note: I used to make my own almond flour by processing blanched almonds in my food processor, which produced marginally acceptable results. Since I started using commercially ground almond flour, my cakes and baked items have been elevated to an entirely different level because of the even, fine texture that I couldn't duplicate. However, I was unable to find a fresh and reliable local supply. I did some research and located a California almond grower who grinds it to order for us, and I make this excellent product available on my website, www.BariatricEating.com.

In addition, while shopping at the mall, I picked up a sunflower baking pan from Williams-Sonoma. It has transformed this plain sponge layer into the most beautiful sculpted cake you can imagine. I present the cake on a platter with decorative bowls of strawberries and cream. After the ooh's and ahh's subside, I cut a wedge of this lovely golden sunflower and assemble each serving in a small dessert bowl (see Sources, page 303).

tangerine custard cakes

Full portion: Calories 130, fat 9 gr, carbs 7 gr, protein 5 gr
Makes six ½-cup servings

This light, tart dessert is the epitome of freshness and summer. Any citrus can be used for this tangy dessert. Sometimes I find fresh Key limes in the market and will either use them solo or combine them with other fresh citrus flavors, but common limes,

lemons, tangelos, and tangerines all add a tart flavor. The dusting
of confectioners' sugar adds minimal sugar carbs but does make
the dessert special, so I splurge without any danger of crossing
the line into the dumping zone. This dessert also works well
baked in a 1½-quart soufflé dish; increase the baking time by
5 minutes.

**3 tablespoons salted butter, at room temperature, plus additional
     for the ramekins**
⅔ cup Splenda Granular
Pinch of salt
3 large eggs, separated
3 tablespoons all-purpose flour
1 cup 2% low-fat milk
**2 tablespoons freshly grated tangerine zest plus 4 tablespoons
     fresh tangerine juice, about 2 small tangerines**
2 tablespoons fresh lemon juice
2 teaspoons confectioners' sugar

Preheat the oven to 325°F. Butter six ½-cup ramekins and place
inside a large roasting pan. Using an electric mixer, blend together
the butter, Splenda, and salt until creamy and smooth. Mix in the egg
yolks. Add the flour and milk and beat until well blended. Stir in the
tangerine zest, tangerine juice, and lemon juice. Beat the egg whites
in a deep bowl with clean beaters until stiff peaks form. Gently fold
one third of the meringue into the batter to lighten, and then fold in
the remaining meringue until well blended. The mixture will have a
somewhat curdled appearance. Spoon the mixture into the prepared
ramekins.

Fill the larger roasting pan with hot water to come halfway up the
sides of the ramekins. Bake for 25 to 30 minutes, until puffed, lightly
browned, and just firm to the touch. Carefully remove the ramekins

from the water to cool. Just before serving, spoon the confectioners' sugar into a fine-mesh sieve and sift over each of the slightly warm custard cakes. This dessert separates into a light spongy soufflé-like layer over a smooth custard layer and is delicious warm or chilled.

raspberry mousse pie

Full portion: Calories 147, fat 12 gr, carbs 8 gr, protein 2 gr
Serves 10

An intense berry puree whipped into a creamy fruit mousse.
This pie is a beautiful shade of soft pink. I have made it with
blackberries and strawberries, but when I use plump raspberries,
I get the most applause. I am a raspberry fiend, and a small slice
of this soft creamy mousse pie is the kind of dessert I dream of.

1 cup Joseph's sugar-free lemon cookies (see Note, page 239)
1 tablespoon salted butter, softened
1 pint fresh raspberries, blackberries, or strawberries
1¼ cups Splenda Granular
1 teaspoon unflavored gelatin (about ⅓ packet)
¼ teaspoon freshly grated lemon zest
½ teaspoon fresh lemon juice
¼ pound reduced-fat cream cheese
1 cup heavy cream

Preheat the oven to 300°F. Finely crush the cookies or pulse in a food processor; blend with the softened butter and evenly press the mixture into a 9-inch pie plate. Bake for 10 minutes and set aside to cool.

Puree 1½ cups of the berries with 1 cup of the Splenda in a food processor or blender. Pass the mixture through a fine-mesh sieve, pressing on the solids to extract as much juice and pulp as possible. Sprinkle the gelatin over 1 tablespoon cold water in a small cup and set aside for 2 minutes without stirring. Warm the berry puree in a small saucepan over medium-low heat, add the softened gelatin, and stir until the gelatin is completely dissolved. Pour into a measuring cup and add water to the berry puree, if necessary, to bring to ¾ cup total. Stir the lemon zest and juice into the puree. Beat the cream cheese in an electric mixer until fluffy; slowly add the berry mixture and beat until smooth. In a separate bowl, blend the heavy cream with the remaining ¼ cup Splenda and whip until medium peaks form. Gently fold half of the whipped cream into the berry mixture to lighten; fold in the rest of the whipped cream and the remaining ½ cup whole berries, and spread the filling in the pie shell. Chill for at least 2 hours before serving.

lemon meringue pie

Full portion: Calories 128, fat 8 gr, carbs 10.5 gr, protein 3.5 gr
Serves 10

A lemon lover's classic and my father's very favorite dessert. He can't tell that this version is sugar-free and it just tickles me to see him taste it and try to detect if I am tricking him. The absence of sugar in the meringue keeps the whites from achieving a deep golden brown when baked, but a carefully watched minute under the broiler is a quick remedy.

1 cup Joseph's sugar-free lemon cookies (see Note, page 239)
1 tablespoon salted butter, melted
1½ cups Splenda Granular
¼ cup cornstarch

¼ teaspoon table salt

3 large eggs, separated, at room temperature

½ cup fresh lemon juice (about 4 lemons)

2 tablespoons butter

1 tablespoon freshly grated lemon zest

3 large egg whites, at room temperature

¼ teaspoon cream of tartar

½ teaspoon vanilla extract

Preheat the oven to 300°F. Finely crush the cookies or pulse in a food processor; blend with the softened butter and evenly press the mixture into a 9-inch pie plate. Bake for 10 minutes and set aside to cool.

Combine 1 cup of the Splenda, the cornstarch, and salt in a medium saucepan. Whisk in 1½ cups cold water. Cook over medium heat, stirring constantly, until the mixture comes to a boil. Reduce the heat to medium-low; continue cooking for 1 minute while the mixture thickens. Remove from the heat.

Whisk the egg yolks in a medium bowl to blend. Slowly whisk about a third of the hot mixture into the egg yolks, then whisk the egg mixture back into the saucepan. Return the pan to medium heat. Cook, stirring constantly, for 2 minutes, until the mixture is smooth and thick. Stir in the lemon juice, butter, and lemon zest, if using, and pour into the baked crust.

Preheat the oven to 275°F. Using an electric mixer, beat the 6 egg whites and the cream of tartar until frothy. Add the vanilla, then gradually beat in the remaining ½ cup Splenda, continuing until stiff peaks form. Mound the meringue on top of the warm lemon filling, spreading it to the crust edges to seal. Bake for 35 to 40 minutes, until the meringue is pale gold. Preheat the broiler and broil for 1 minute, watching constantly, until the meringue is browned. Cool to room temperature and chill before serving.

toasted coconut custards

Full portion: Calories 125, fat 8 gr, carbs 8 gr, protein 6 gr
Serves 8

A perfect coconut-flavored, smooth custard that is delicious
baked in a pie shell or in individual ramekins. I bake my ceramic
ramekins in a water bath for 30 minutes, or until the center jiggles
just a bit, and serve chilled.

Unsalted butter
3 ounces unsweetened coconut (frozen grated coconut is
    excellent; you can find it in the frozen fruits section)
3 large eggs
1 cup Splenda Granular
2 teaspoons coconut extract
1 teaspoon vanilla extract
3 cups 2% low-fat milk
½ cup unsweetened coconut milk

Preheat the oven to 325°F. Lightly butter a 2-inch-deep 8 × 10–inch
or 1½-quart round baking dish and place inside a large roasting pan.
Spread the coconut on a baking sheet and bake until lightly toasted
and golden in color, about 15 minutes.

Beat the eggs in a deep bowl until frothy and lemon-colored.
Gradually whisk in the Splenda until well blended. Stir in the coconut extract, vanilla, milk, coconut milk, and toasted coconut. Pour
the mixture into the prepared baking dish. Fill the roasting pan with
hot water to come halfway up the sides of the baking dish. Bake for
35 to 40 minutes, until the center is still a bit soft. Carefully remove
the baking dish from the water and let cool. Serve warm or chilled.

crepes suzette

Per crepe: Calories 67, fat 2.5 gr, carbs 6.5 gr, protein 2.5 gr
Makes 8 to 10 crepes

Make the crepes a day in advance if you wish—just stack, wrap
in plastic, and refrigerate. The recipe also can be easily doubled
or tripled to accommodate your number of guests. I usually serve
two crepes per person for a light finish.

2 large eggs
½ cup skim milk
Pinch of table salt
2 tablespoons Splenda Granular
1 teaspoon vanilla extract
½ cup all-purpose flour
Vegetable oil cooking spray
1 tablespoon salted butter
¼ cup Nature's Hollow Apricot Preserves
Zest and juice of 1 orange
¼ cup Grand Marnier or light rum
Whipped cream sweetened to taste with Splenda, optional

Whisk together the eggs and milk in a large bowl. Blend in the salt,
Splenda, vanilla, and flour. Set aside for 30 minutes.

Spray a nonstick 8-inch skillet or omelet pan with cooking spray
and heat over medium heat. Ladle 2 tablespoons of the batter into the
center of the pan. Lift the pan from the burner and swirl the pan so
the batter smoothly coats the entire bottom. Replace the pan on the
burner and cook just until the batter looks dry. Flip the crepe, using a
spatula or your fingers, and cook the other side for 10 to 15 seconds.

Transfer to a plate. Repeat until the batter is used up, lightly coating the pan with the cooking spray between crepes.

Melt together the butter, preserves, orange zest, orange juice, and Grand Marnier in a large nonstick skillet over medium-high heat; gently simmer until the mixture comes together in a light syrup.

Working quickly, take the first crepe and dip one side into the warm syrup; fold in half, syrup side in, and then fold again into quarters. Stack each of the folded crepes to one side of the pan while you prepare the rest. When all the crepes are folded, arrange them evenly in the pan and gently warm them in the sauce over medium-high heat for 1 minute, carefully turning each crepe to completely coat. Place two of the warm, folded crepes on each plate, spoon on some of the sauce, and top with a little Splenda-sweetened whipped cream, if desired.

chocolate cream crepes

Per crepe: Calories 57, fat 1.5 gr, carbs 8 gr, protein 3 gr
Makes 8 to 10 crepes

I use my prettiest dessert plates and serve two delicate but richly flavored chocolate crepes rolled up around a filling of chocolate whipped cream and a few fresh raspberries, lightly dusted with cocoa and confectioners' sugar. You can get very creative with your choice of fillings but keep the carbohydrate count anchored in reality.

2 large eggs
½ cup plus 2 tablespoons skim milk
Pinch of table salt
2 tablespoons Splenda Granular

1 teaspoon vanilla extract

2 tablespoons plus 1 teaspoon Dutch-processed cocoa

½ cup all-purpose flour

Vegetable oil cooking spray

Chocolate Reddi-wip, or 1 cup heavy cream, whipped and
sweetened with Splenda and cocoa

1 teaspoon confectioners' sugar

Fresh raspberries or strawberries

Whisk together the eggs and milk in a large bowl. Blend in the salt, Splenda, vanilla, 2 tablespoons of the cocoa, and the flour. Set the batter aside for 30 minutes.

Spray a nonstick 8-inch skillet or omelet pan with the nonstick cooking spray and heat over medium heat. Ladle 2 tablespoons of the batter into the center of the pan. Lift the pan from the burner and swirl the pan so the batter smoothly coats the entire bottom. Replace the pan on the burner and cook just until the batter looks dry. Flip the crepe, using a spatula or your fingers, and cook the other side for 10 to 15 seconds. Transfer to a plate. Repeat until the batter is used up, lightly coating the pan with the nonstick spray between crepes.

Place 1 crepe on a plate, make a thick line of chocolate cream down the center, and roll. Repeat with the remaining crepes. Place 2 rolled crepes on each of 4 plates. Spoon the remaining teaspoon of cocoa powder and the confectioners' sugar side by side into a fine-mesh strainer and tap over the crepes to dust. Place the berries on the plate and serve immediately.

cream puffs

Per puff: Calories 74, fat 6.5 gr, carbs 2.5 gr,
protein 1 gr
Makes twenty-four 2-inch cream puffs

This is a very simple dessert, and well worth the time it takes to properly prepare the puff shells. Using a food processor makes this a snap, as it takes strong arms to beat the dough without one. Resist the urge to pipe large mounds on the baking sheet, as they double during baking. Make them about the size of a cherry tomato for perfect three-to-a-serving cream puffs. Even though it is a bit unconventional, whipping the instant pudding mix with the heavy cream stabilizes the mixture and sweetens it as well. It is a delicious filling so don't discount it just because it uses instant pudding mix. The puffs can also be filled with small scoops of no-sugar-added ice milk and drizzled with melted sugar-free chocolate.

Vegetable oil cooking spray
2 large eggs
1 large egg white
5 tablespoons salted butter
2 tablespoons 1% low-fat milk
2 teaspoons Splenda Granular
Pinch of table salt
½ cup all-purpose flour
1 tablespoon Jell-O Sugar-Free Instant Vanilla Pudding mix
1 cup heavy cream
1 teaspoon vanilla extract
Confectioners' sugar

Preheat the oven to 425°F. Lightly spray a large baking sheet with cooking spray. Lightly beat the eggs and egg white in a glass measuring cup; discard any excess over ½ cup and set aside.

In a medium saucepan over medium-high heat, bring the butter, milk, ¼ cup plus 2 tablespoons water, Splenda, and salt to a boil. When the mixture reaches a full boil, remove from the heat and stir in the flour with a wooden spoon until combined and the mixture pulls away from the sides of the pan. Return the saucepan to low heat and cook, stirring constantly using a smearing motion, for 3 minutes, until the mixture is shiny and smooth.

Transfer the mixture to a food processor and process for a few seconds with the feed tube open to cool the mixture slightly. With the machine running, add the eggs in a steady stream, scrape down the sides of the bowl, then process for 30 seconds or until a smooth, sticky paste forms. Scrape the mixture into a large plastic bag, push the paste into the bottom of the bag, and cut off one corner about ½ inch from the tip to use as a pastry bag (or use a pastry bag if you have one).

Pipe the paste into 1-inch mounds on the baking sheet. Lightly smooth the surface of each mound using a fingertip dipped in water. Bake for 15 minutes, reduce the oven temperature to 375°F, and continue to bake 8 to 10 minutes longer, until golden brown.

Remove the baking sheet from the oven. With the tip of a small knife, cut a tiny slit into the side of each puff to release the steam, and return the puffs to the oven. Turn the oven off and, leaving the door ajar, dry the puffs in the oven for about 45 minutes. Remove from the oven, and when cool, store in an airtight container or plastic bag.

Place the pudding powder in a small deep bowl, add the cream and vanilla, and beat with a handheld mixer past the soft peak stage until the mixture gets very smooth and thick, about 3 minutes. Scrape the mixture into a large plastic bag, push it into the bottom of the bag, and cut off a corner about ⅓ inch from the tip. Just before serving, slice the puffs with a serrated knife, fill the bottoms with a swirl of the vanilla cream, and replace the tops. Dust with confectioners' sugar and serve immediately.

strawberry fool

Full portion: Calories 179, fat 15 gr, carbs 11.5 gr, protein 1.5 gr
Makes six ½-cup servings

This pudding captures the essence of fresh berries. I serve this dessert in a beautiful stemmed wineglass and spear a giant, whole, perfect berry on the edge of the glass for a dramatic presentation.

1 quart ripe strawberries, rinsed and hulled,
   6 reserved for presentation
¼ cup Nature's Hollow Strawberry Preserves
2 tablespoons Splenda Granular
Pinch of freshly grated nutmeg
½ teaspoon vanilla extract
1 cup heavy cream

Coarsely chop half of the berries and place in a small saucepan with the preserves and Splenda. Heat over medium-high heat until the berries begin to release juice and the preserves have dissolved, about 2 minutes. Transfer to a large bowl; stir in the nutmeg and vanilla, and chill. Slice the remaining strawberries and set aside. When ready to serve, whip the cream to stiff peaks. Stir the sliced strawberries into the cooled strawberry mixture and gently fold in the whipped cream, half at a time. Spoon into serving dishes and garnish with the reserved whole berries.

walker's favorite chocolate pudding

Full portion: Calories 42, fat .5 gr, carbs 10 gr, protein 1 gr
Makes six ½-cup servings

One weekend I was experimenting with chocolate protein pudding recipes and it so happened that Ronni's sister Victoria and three-year-old niece, Walker, were visiting from Seattle. At this particular time the mainstays of Walker's diet were bacon and chocolate pudding, so I obviously couldn't have dreamed of finding anyone better suited to judge which of the three versions was tastiest. I took my three bowls of pudding to Grandma Joyce's house, and we had an old-fashioned taste test. This one was, without a doubt, Walker's favorite. Upon turning four she stopped eating bacon after discovering to her horror that it comes from pigs.

One 12-ounce package silken tofu
2 teaspoons vanilla extract
⅓ cup Splenda Granular
3 ounces sugar-free chocolate, preferably Valor or Guylian
Heavy cream, softly whipped and lightly sweetened with
    Splenda Granular

Puree the tofu, vanilla, and Splenda in a blender until smooth and custard-like, scraping down the sides as necessary. Break the chocolate into pieces and melt in a small bowl in the microwave: heat on high for 45 to 60 seconds, until just melted. Add the melted chocolate to the tofu mixture; pulse until well blended and smooth. Pour into 6 individual dessert ramekins and chill. Serve with a swirl of whipped cream.

cannoli pudding

Full portion: Calories 123, fat 8 gr, carbs 6 gr, protein 8 gr
Serves 8

Once again the Italian in me comes to the surface. One of my "last meals" before my bariatric surgery consisted of anchovy pizza, with two cannolis for dessert. Little did I know that after my surgery I would be making cannoli cream that was indistinguishable from the full-sugar filling I have made for years. You must use a food processor to get the smooth custard consistency, because ricotta has a grainy texture that does not translate well into a pudding. This dessert should be assembled just before serving, or the pistachios will lose their crispness. Once you have shelled the pistachios, roll the nuts in a tea towel to remove the papery coating.

One 15-ounce container part-skim ricotta cheese
⅔ cup Splenda Granular
1 teaspoon vanilla extract
1 tablespoon sugar-free instant vanilla pudding powder
About 1 ounce sugar-free chocolate, such as Valor or Guylian,
     shaved (see Note, page 241)
½ cup coarsely chopped shelled pistachio nuts

Puree the ricotta with the Splenda, vanilla, and pudding powder in a food processor until smooth and creamy. Transfer the mixture to a medium bowl and chill before serving. Place a swirl of the cannoli cream into a martini glass or small dessert dish and sprinkle liberally with the shaved chocolate and chopped pistachios; serve immediately.

fresh blueberries
with vanilla crème anglaise

Full portion: Calories 98, fat 3 gr, carbs 12 gr, protein 5 gr
Makes four ½-cup servings

A great dessert for a hot day or after a comfort-food meal when you want just a little something sweet and refreshing. This vanilla custard sauce is delicious with any fresh ripe seasonal fruit—raspberries, kiwi, mango, blackberries, or strawberries are all perfect for this presentation. Just watch the carbohydrate count of your fruit selections to keep this dessert light; don't use more than a half cup of fruit. Garnish this dessert with a single sugar-free butter cookie.

1½ cups 1% low-fat milk
Pinch of table salt
½ cup Splenda Granular
3 large egg yolks
1½ teaspoons vanilla extract
1 pint fresh blueberries, washed and drained

Whisk together the milk, salt, and ¼ cup of the Splenda in a medium saucepan. Bring the mixture just to the simmering point over medium heat. Combine the egg yolks with the remaining ¼ cup Splenda in a medium bowl and, whisking constantly, slowly pour in half of the hot milk mixture, blending until smooth. Pour the egg mixture into the saucepan, whisking until well combined. Place the saucepan over medium heat and stir constantly until the custard is thick enough to coat the back of a spoon, 5 to 6 minutes; it should never boil. Strain into a bowl and stir in the vanilla. Let cool slightly. Place plastic wrap directly on the surface of the custard and chill before serving.

To serve, pile ½ cup of the blueberries in the center of each martini glass or dessert dish and pour the chilled cream around the berries.

coffee panna cotta

Full portion: Calories 102, fat 1.5 gr, carbs 12 gr, protein 9 gr
Makes six ½-cup servings

A quivering dish of coffee-infused cream. Add a tablespoon of DaVinci Sugar-Free Hazelnut Syrup (see Sources, page 303) for a pudding version of your favorite latte.

2 teaspoons unflavored gelatin (about ⅔ packet)
2 cups evaporated low-fat milk
1¼ cups 1% low-fat milk
1 tablespoon vanilla extract
3 tablespoons ground coffee
½ cup Splenda Granula
Whipped cream sweetened with Splenda
Ground cinnamon

Sprinkle the gelatin over 2 tablespoons of cold water in a small cup and let soak for 3 minutes without stirring. Heat the milks, vanilla, coffee, and Splenda over medium-high heat, stirring occasionally. As soon as the mixture starts to boil, remove the pan from the heat and add the gelatin mixture, stirring to completely dissolve the gelatin. Strain the mixture through a very-fine-mesh strainer into a large measuring cup. If necessary, strain the mixture several times to remove all of the coffee grounds, rinsing the strainer each time and allowing the mixture to settle before pouring. Pour into 6 ramekins or dessert cups. Chill 6 to 8 hours, until set.

To serve, run the tip of a knife around the edge of the custard, dip the ramekin almost to the rim into a bowl of very hot water for 15 seconds, cover with a dessert plate, and flip. Serve with a dollop of softly whipped cream to the side and lightly dust the entire dessert with ground cinnamon.

orange panna cotta
with berry coulis

Full portion: Calories 110, fat 2 gr, carbs 15 gr, protein 8 gr
Makes four ½-cup servings

The tartness of the yogurt, the freshness of the orange zest, and the bright flavor of the strawberry sauce make this dessert a standout. Traditional panna cotta is a flavored cream thickened with gelatin, but this version has an unexpected burst of citrus. This dessert makes a nice presentation for a special occasion. I have little heart-shaped ramekins that I found at a discount store, and the white custard heart is beautifully contrasted by the strawberry sauce.

If you don't already have one, microplane graters are fabulous and this dessert gives you an excuse to buy one. One of these indispensable, super-sharp graters turns orange peel into a pile of golden gossamer threads that really infuse the custard with flavor.

1 pint (16 ounces) vanilla low-fat yogurt sweetened with Splenda or Equal, such as Blue Bunny Lite 85 or Dannon Light & Fit
⅓ cup Splenda Granular
1½ teaspoons vanilla extract
1 teaspoon freshly grated orange zest, lightly packed
2 teaspoons unflavored gelatin (about ⅔ packet)
5 tablespoons fresh orange juice
1 cup fresh strawberries (or unsweetened frozen strawberries)
2 tablespoons Nature's Hollow Strawberry Preserves

In a large bowl, whisk together the yogurt, Splenda, vanilla, and orange zest. In a very small saucepan, sprinkle the gelatin over 3 tablespoons of the orange juice and let stand undisturbed for 1 minute to soften. Warm the mixture over low heat until the gelatin has completely dissolved. Whisk the warm gelatin into the yogurt mixture and pour into 4 ramekins or custard cups. Chill the panna cotta at least 6 to 8 hours, until firm.

Place the berries, the remaining 2 tablespoons of orange juice, and the preserves in a food processor or blender and process until smooth, adding a little more orange juice if needed to make a puree. Cover and chill the sauce.

To serve, run a thin knife around the edge of each panna cotta; dip the ramekin, almost to the rim, into a bowl of very hot water for 15 seconds; cover with a dessert plate; and flip. Pour some of the berry coulis around each custard and serve immediately.

fresh cherry clafouti

Full portion: Calories 82, fat 2 gr, carbs 8 gr, protein 5 gr
Serves 10

This dessert is an amazing combination of fluffy, almond-flavored
custard and sweet ripe cherries. The biggest, darkest fresh
cherries are best for the ultimate flavor, but frozen cherries work
well in a pinch if you drop them into the batter while they're still
frozen. If you can't find cherries in the market, fresh or frozen
blueberries will also make your mouth water. Once again, the
light dusting of confectioners' sugar will only add a gram or
two of sugar to the entire dessert, but really adds a spectacular
finishing touch.

½ cup 1% low-fat milk
½ cup part-skim ricotta cheese
2 large eggs
½ cup Splenda Granular
½ cup all-purpose flour
½ teaspoon vanilla extract
½ teaspoon almond extract
Vegetable oil cooking spray
1 cup fresh pitted cherries
Confectioners' sugar

Preheat the oven to 425°F. Combine the milk, ricotta, eggs, Splenda,
flour, vanilla, and almond extract in a food processor or blender,
blending until smooth. Let the batter rest for 20 minutes.

Lightly spray the bottom of a 9-inch round ceramic baking dish
with cooking spray. Pour the batter into the dish and evenly arrange

the cherries in the batter. Bake for 30 to 35 minutes, until puffed and golden brown. Serve warm cut into wedges, and dust with confectioners' sugar.

spiced pumpkin custard

Full portion: Calories 84, fat 3 gr, carbs 8 gr, protein 6 gr
Makes eight ½-cup servings

Served warm with a dollop of whipped cream, this cinnamon- and ginger-flecked, creamy pumpkin custard is an anytime favorite. It can also be an excellent addition to a holiday table, and it is a great dessert to cart along to a family member's house so you can avoid the full-sugar pumpkin pie that is sure to be there.

Vegetable oil cooking spray
¾ cup Splenda Granular
½ teaspoon table salt
1 teaspoon ground cinnamon
½ teaspoon ground ginger
¼ teaspoon ground cloves
3 large eggs
One 15-ounce can Libby's 100% Pure Pumpkin (not pumpkin pie filling)
One 12-ounce can evaporated low-fat milk (not sweetened condensed milk)
Whipped cream sweetened with Splenda, or Reddi-wip

Preheat the oven to 325°F. Lightly spray eight ½-cup ramekins or custard cups with vegetable cooking spray and place in a large roasting pan.

Mix the Splenda, salt, cinnamon, ginger, and cloves in a small bowl. Beat the eggs in a large bowl. Blend in the pumpkin and the spice mixture. Gradually blend in the evaporated milk.

Ladle the filling into the prepared ramekins. Pour very hot water into the roasting pan to come about halfway up the sides of the ramekins.

Bake for 25 to 30 minutes, or until a thin knife inserted near the center of the custard comes out clean. Carefully remove the ramekins from the hot water. Serve warm or chilled. Top with Splenda-sweetened whipped cream or a squirt of Reddi-wip before serving, if desired.

light banana bread

WLS portion (1 slice): Calories 97, fat 6 gr, carbs 7 gr, protein 3 gr
Makes 1 loaf (16 slices)

This is an improved version of my original recipe, which replaces the Splenda and protein powder with fresh California almond flour and Truvia Baking Blend. This superb sugar replacer makes a delicious, healthy loaf that is indistinguishable from a full-sugar, full-fat version. Cut in half and freeze a portion of this loaf, or wrap individual slices. Make sure you measure the mashed banana accurately, as almond flour does not absorb moisture and your bread will be too wet if you add too much banana.

Vegetable oil cooking spray
1 cup mashed ripe banana, about 2 medium bananas
1 teaspoon vanilla extract

1 large egg
½ cup Truvia Baking Blend
½ cup all-purpose flour
1 cup almond flour (see Note, page 246)
2½ teaspoons baking powder
¼ teaspoon salt
2 tablespoons butter, melted
⅔ cup chopped pecans or walnuts

Preheat the oven to 350°F. Lightly spray a 9 × 5 × 3–inch loaf pan with cooking spray.

Combine the bananas, vanilla, egg, and Truvia in a large bowl. Mix the flours, baking powder, and salt in a small bowl, then add to the wet ingredients, gently folding to incorporate. Stir in the butter and pecans. Pour the batter into the prepared loaf pan and bake for 40 to 50 minutes, until a toothpick inserted into the center comes out clean. Cool in the pan on a rack for 10 minutes, remove, and cool before slicing.

almond-anise biscotti

Per cookie: Calories 90, fat 8 gr, carbs 2.5 gr, protein 1 gr
Makes 2 dozen cookies

One of my nicest memories is of the many large tins of delicious biscotti my grandmother and her sister Lena baked at Christmas. When I started experimenting with almond flour, traditional Italian biscotti came to mind immediately, since most recipes already have almond extract and whole almonds in the dough. The result is amazing: toasted almonds, mild anise flavor, and the nuttiness of the almond flour—tough to believe it is sugar-free as well.

To really put these biscotti over the top, melt half a bar of Valor Sugar-Free Spanish Dark chocolate in a shallow bowl in the microwave (45 to 60 seconds on high, then stir with a fork until melted) and dip the bottom of each biscotti, allowing the chocolate to come about one third of the way up the sides. Place the dipped biscotti on a wax paper–lined baking sheet and pop the baking sheet into the freezer. When the chocolate is hard, transfer the cookies to an airtight container.

1 large egg

1 large egg white

1 cup Splenda Granular

2 tablespoons salted butter, melted

2 teaspoons vanilla extract

2 teaspoons freshly ground anise seed (see Note), or ½ teaspoon
    anise extract

2 cups almond flour (see Note, page 246)

½ cup all-purpose flour

1½ teaspoons baking powder

Pinch of table salt

½ cup whole blanched almonds, toasted on a baking sheet at
    350°F until lightly golden

Vegetable oil cooking spray

Using an electric mixer, beat the egg and egg white until thick and lemon-colored. Add the Splenda, butter, vanilla, and ground anise, and continue beating until well blended. Mix the almond flour, all-purpose flour, baking powder, and salt in a small bowl. Add to the egg mixture and stir until well blended. Give a few rough chops to the toasted almonds with a heavy knife, and fold them into the dough. Cover and refrigerate for 20 minutes to firm the dough for handling.

Preheat the oven to 350°F. Turn the dough out onto wax paper that has been lightly sprayed with cooking spray and, using the paper, roll the dough into a 12-inch-long by 2-inch-wide flattened log shape. Transfer to a baking sheet by picking up the paper and rolling the biscotti log onto the sheet. Bake for 35 to 40 minutes, until golden brown and firm to the touch. Cool completely on the baking sheet. Carefully remove the biscotti log to a cutting board and, using a serrated knife, cut into ½-inch-thick slices. Arrange the slices on the same baking sheet. Bake for 14 minutes at 350°F; turn the biscotti over and bake for an additional 8 to 10 minutes, until golden brown. Cool and store in an airtight container.

Note: I have a small electric coffee grinder that I use just for spices.

strawberry italian ice

Full portion: Calories 42, fat .5 gr, carbs 10 gr, protein 1 gr
Makes six ½-cup servings

This dessert is simple, fresh, and fruity, with a hint of blended citrus. Substitute any unsweetened berry, or even fresh-frozen mango cubes, for the strawberries; just use lower-carbohydrate fruits. Make a double batch for a backyard barbecue or outdoor party. The citrus syrup may be prepared in advance and refrigerated. It is also delicious as a sweetener and flavoring for iced tea.

One 16-ounce package frozen whole unsweetened strawberries
Zest and juice of 1 orange (about ⅓ cup juice)
Zest and juice of 1 lemon (about 2 tablespoons juice)
1 cup Splenda Granular

Slightly thaw the strawberries by placing them in a large bowl at room temperature while the other components are being prepared, about 20 minutes.

Remove wide strips of zest from the orange and lemon with a vegetable peeler and scrape off any bitter white pith. Combine the Splenda with ½ cup water in a small saucepan and add the citrus zests and juices. Bring the mixture to a boil, reduce the heat, and simmer for 5 minutes. Allow the syrup to cool a bit, and then strain the mixture, discarding the zests.

Transfer the strawberries to a food processor or blender, add ½ cup of the citrus syrup, and pulse until a nearly smooth, frosty puree is formed, adding more syrup to blend, if necessary. Transfer the semi-frozen puree to a bowl and freeze for 2 to 3 hours, until firm.

To serve, let stand at room temperature for 15 to 20 minutes to soften slightly, scrape across the Italian ice with a large spoon, and place into serving dishes.

lemon bars

Per each 2-inch square: Calories 73, fat 5 gr, carbs 4 gr, protein 2 gr
Makes twenty-four 2-inch squares

I love lemon, and this is a delicious no-sugar version that is perfect to take to a holiday office party or family barbecue. Very tart with a buttery crust!

Vegetable oil cooking spray
¾ cup plus 3 tablespoons all-purpose flour
¾ cup almond flour (see Note, page 246)

1½ cups Truvia Baking Blend, plus more for dusting

6 tablespoons (¾ stick) salted butter

½ teaspoon baking powder

½ teaspoon table salt

1 teaspoon grated lemon zest

⅔ cup fresh lemon juice (about 3 lemons)

4 large eggs

Preheat the oven to 350°F and lightly coat an 8½ × 11–inch oblong pan with cooking spray.

Pulse ¾ cup of all-purpose flour, ¾ cup of almond flour, ½ cup Truvia, and butter in the food processor until the mixture resembles coarse meal. Press into the prepared pan and bake for 18 to 20 minutes, until the crust is golden and firm to the touch.

Combine the remaining cup of Truvia, 3 tablespoons flour, baking powder, and salt in a medium bowl. Add the lemon zest and juice and eggs, whisking until smooth. Pour the mixture over the crust. Bake for 14 to 16 minutes, until set. Remove from the oven; cool in the pan on a wire rack. Cut into 24 squares. Dust with additional Truvia just before serving.

almond macaroons

Per cookie: Calories 36, fat 3 gr, carbs 1.5 gr, protein 1.5 gr
Makes 36 cookies

Chewy, moist, and delicious; a wonderful cookie that happens to be sugar-free. These will become a family favorite as they are fabulously simple and taste superb. Make life easier and invest in a roll of parchment paper to line your baking sheet; it makes a huge difference. I use a one-tablespoon metal ice-cream scoop for measuring an even portion for perfect batches of cookies.

½ cup Truvia Baking Blend
¼ cup all-purpose flour
4 tablespoons (½ stick) butter, melted
1 egg white, slightly beaten
½ teaspoon vanilla extract
2¼ cups sliced unblanched almonds, about 10 ounces
½ cup dried cranberries, also called craisins

Cover a baking sheet with a piece of parchment paper, and set aside. Preheat the oven to 350°F.

Combine the Truvia, flour, butter, egg white, and vanilla in a large bowl; add the almonds and cranberries, then toss well to evenly moisten the mixture. Mound tablespoonfuls of the mixture on the prepared baking sheet. Bake for 10 to 12 minutes, until golden. Cool completely before moving to a baking rack. Store in an airtight container.

pistachio gelato

WLS ⅓-cup serving: Calories 67, fat 2 gr, carbs 7 gr, protein 3 gr
Makes 4 cups

When I traveled to Tuscany with my aunt Gail in 2006, we were amused by the number of slim Italians crowded around gelato shops on every corner in every town we passed through. In Italy, gelato is served in tiny cups and eaten with tiny scoops; quality and moderation seem to be the rule. Gail is a diabetic, and I of course can't eat sugar, so we were on a quest to find a *gelato artigianale* that served a handmade sugar-free gelato. We found just one tiny shop on a corner in Florence, and the sugar-free chocolate and pistachio we savored are as much a part of our memory as the gold on Ponte Vecchio and the magnificence of David.

I plug in my Cuisinart automatic ice-cream machine, get the metal insert from my freezer, pour in the chilled custard, and in 30 minutes I am eating a small cup of outrageous homemade pistachio gelato that takes me back to Italy!

3 cups fat-free half-and-half
1 cup shelled pistachio nuts
1 ¼ cups Splenda Granular
1 teaspoon almond extract
1 teaspoon vanilla extract

Puree the half-and-half, pistachios, Splenda, and almond and vanilla extracts in a blender until you have a smooth, pale green liquid. Refrigerate the mixture until cold, about 3 hours or preferably overnight. Process the custard in an ice-cream maker according to the manufacturer's instructions. Transfer to a covered container and freeze.

strawberry jelly roll

One slice: Calories 52, fat 2 gr, carbs 9 gr, protein 3 gr
Makes twelve ¾-inch slices

Everyone loves a jelly roll, and they look marvelous in the center of a beautiful decorative platter. Fold any flavor of sugar-free preserves or Splenda-sweetened fresh fruit puree into whipped cream to vary the fillings and you can use this recipe as your signature sugar-free dessert! One of my favorite combinations uses 1 cup of well-drained Libby's Splenda-sweetened crushed pineapple, folded into 2 tablespoons of Jell-O Sugar-Free instant Vanilla Pudding powder whipped with 1 cup heavy cream.

Vegetable oil cooking spray
5 large eggs, separated
½ cup Truvia Baking Blend, plus more for dusting
1 teaspoon vanilla extract
½ cup all-purpose flour
1 cup Nature's Hollow Sugar-Free Strawberry Preserves

Preheat the oven to 350°F. Coat a 15 × 10 × 1–inch baking sheet with cooking spray and line with a piece of wax paper; lightly coat the paper with cooking spray.

Beat the egg whites in a large bowl with electric beaters until soft peaks form. Add ¼ cup of the Truvia, a little at a time, and beat until stiff, glossy peaks form when the beaters are lifted. Do not overbeat.

In a small bowl, beat the egg yolks with the remaining ¼ cup Truvia and the vanilla until very thick, 7 to 8 minutes. Using low speed, beat in the flour until blended. With a rubber spatula, gently fold the egg-yolk mixture into the beaten whites just until blended.

Spread the batter in the prepared pan. Bake for 10 to 12 minutes, until the cake springs back when lightly pressed.

Run a thin knife around the pan edges to loosen the cake. Slide the wax paper and the cake from the pan onto a clean kitchen towel and allow to cool. Using the wax paper as a guide, flip the cake onto the towel so the paper side is up and carefully peel the paper from the cake.

Spread the jam evenly over the cake. Starting from a short side, roll the cake using the towel to push and roll firmly. Place the rolled cake seam side down on a platter and lightly dust with Truvia.

rich chocolate cake

Full portion: Calories 159, fat 11 g, carbs 10 g, protein 4 g
Serves 10

Sometimes you need a perfectly moist single round layer for a party or special event; the kind of cake that needs a dollop of real whipped cream and nothing else. I decided to make the focus of this cake "sugar-free," and not substitute almond flour to reduce carbohydrates. It is delicious, dark, and decadent.

Vegetable oil cooking spray
1 cup all-purpose flour
½ cup unsweetened cocoa
1 teaspoon baking powder
½ teaspoon baking soda
¼ teaspoon salt
½ cup (1 stick) butter, softened
1 cup Truvia Baking Blend
2 large eggs
1 teaspoon vanilla extract
⅔ cup milk

Preheat the oven to 350°F. Lightly spray an 8-inch round cake pan with vegetable spray. Line the bottom with a round of wax paper and spray again.

In a medium bowl, combine the flour, cocoa, baking powder,

baking soda, and salt. In a large bowl, beat the butter and Truvia using a mixer at high speed; continue to beat until light and fluffy, 3 to 4 minutes. Add the eggs one at a time, beating well after each addition. Beat in the vanilla. Reduce the speed to low and add the flour mixture alternately with the milk, beginning and ending with the flour. Beat until the batter is smooth, scraping down the bowl with a rubber spatula.

Pour the batter into the prepared pan. Bake for 30 to 35 minutes, until a toothpick inserted in the center comes out almost clean. Cool in the pan on a wire rack for 10 minutes; invert the cake onto the rack to cool completely.

sugar-free oatmeal almond granola

WLS portion (¼ cup): Calories 36, fat 3 g, carbs 2 g, protein 1 g
Makes 4 cups

This nutty no-sugar granola is perfect for a little chewy goodness, and the primary ingredient—rolled oats—is a slow-burning *good carbohydrate*. Stir granola, sugar-free Nature's Hollow preserves, and a spoonful of protein into organic or Greek yogurt for a substantial and healthy breakfast. Stir granola into a sugar-free pudding cup or use as a crunchy topping for summer berries. Enjoy a small portion moistened with Splenda-sweetened vanilla soy milk.

You can also bake the mixture into oatmeal almond cookie crisps, which are perfect to take to a holiday party or to nibble with a cup of Matrix warm protein cocoa. Drop the granola mixture by heaping teaspoons onto two parchment-lined baking sheets. Spray the bottom of a small spatula with nonstick cooking spray and flatten each cookie into a 2-inch round, making the edges as even as possible. Bake until the edges are golden brown. Cool completely on the baking sheets. Remove by peeling the parchment away from the cookies.

1 large egg
4 tablespoons (½ stick) butter, melted
1 teaspoon vanilla extract
½ teaspoon ground cinnamon
½ cup Truvia Baking Blend
1¼ cups rolled oats, not instant or quick-cooking
¾ cup sliced almonds
Vegetable oil cooking spray

Preheat the oven to 350°F and line a baking sheet with parchment paper or a silicon nonstick liner. This is an important step, because without a liner, the mixture will adhere to the pan.

Whisk together the egg, butter, vanilla, cinnamon, and Truvia until smooth. Add the oatmeal and almonds; mix well to coat. Press the mixture into a thin solid layer on the prepared baking sheet. Bake for 12 to 14 minutes, until golden; cool and then break into bite-size pieces. Store in an airtight container or resealable plastic bag.

beatrice's apricot
cream cheese cookies

Per cookie: Calories 35, fat 3 gr, carbs 2 gr
Makes about 30 cookies

These sugar-free cookies are from my mother's repertoire of
Italian Christmas cookie recipes. The dough is tender and flaky
and the sweet-tart apricot filling is perfect. Don't let the short
ingredient list throw you; they taste out of this world. Serve with
a warm mug of Matrix protein cocoa for a healthy dessert on a
cold winter night.

4 ounces cream cheese
4 ounces (1 stick) butter
1 cup flour, plus additional for rolling
¼ teaspoon salt
½ cup Nature's Hollow Sugar-Free Apricot Preserves

Blend the cream cheese and butter. Add the flour and salt, then blend
until the flour is completely incorporated. Gather the dough into a
smooth ball, cover with plastic wrap, and chill for 1 to 2 hours.

Preheat the oven to 375°F. Lightly dust the counter with flour
and roll out half of the dough to ⅛ inch thickness. Using a sharp
knife, carefully cut the dough into 2-inch squares, saving scraps to
re-roll. Stir the preserves with a spoon to a smooth consistency.

Place ¼ teaspoon of preserves in the center of each square. Fold
over two opposite corners of the square to the middle, overlapping
slightly and pressing so they stick together and the jam squishes out a
bit. After folding each cookie, transfer to an ungreased baking sheet,
about 1 inch apart.

Bake each batch for 10 to12 minutes, until the bottoms are just barely turning golden brown. Gently press down any overlapped corners that have opened while baking. Transfer to a wire rack. Repeat with the remaining dough.

When the cookies are cool, place an additional small dab of apricot preserves on each side of the folded cookie.

orange sponge cake

Per square: Calories 45, fat 3 gr, carbs 4 gr, protein 2 gr
Makes sixteen 2-inch squares

This cake is perfect for topping with a few sliced sweetened berries and a squirt of whipped cream or Cool Whip, or tasty and moist on its own. Really punch up the citrus flavor by adding fresh orange zest. I love to serve this cake, and it is so easy to make. This cake features Truvia as a contrast to my similar version using Splenda on page 244.

Vegetable oil cooking spray
¾ cup almond flour (see Note, page 246)
½ cup all-purpose flour
1½ teaspoons baking powder
½ teaspoon salt
3 large eggs
¾ cup Truvia Baking Blend
⅓ cup hot water
1 teaspoon vanilla extract
½ teaspoon orange extract

Spray a nonstick 9-inch square or round pan with cooking spray and line with a piece of parchment or wax paper.

Blend the flours, baking powder, and salt. Beat the eggs in a small mixer bowl until very thick and lemon-colored; add the Truvia and continue beating until doubled in volume. Slowly add the hot water, vanilla extract, and orange extract while continuing to beat on low speed. Fold in the dry ingredients until well blended. Pour into the prepared pan. Bake for 20 to 25 minutes, until the cake tests done. Turn out onto a cooling rack and peel off the paper.

sugar-free molten chocolate cakes

Per serving: Calories 273, fat 24 gr, carbs 2 gr, protein 5 gr
Makes 6 individual cakes

This is my trademark dessert as it tastes extraordinary yet is very easy to make. The cakes are every bit as good as any full-sugar version served in a fine restaurant. The rich, dark exterior is only surpassed by the warm fudge interior. The cakes are not low in fat or calories, so they are not an everyday dessert; however, for a special occasion, they will knock everyone's socks off. I serve mine with a small scoop of Breyer's No Sugar Added Ice Cream on the side and a pool of Splenda-sweetened fresh raspberry puree.

Vegetable oil cooking spray
4 tablespoons (½ stick) unsalted butter
5 to 6 ounces imported sugar-free dark chocolate (see Note, page 241)
3 large eggs
1 egg yolk

1 teaspoon vanilla extract
½ cup Splenda Granular
Pinch of table salt
2 tablespoons all-purpose flour

Preheat the oven to 400°F. Lightly spray six 6-ounce ramekins with cooking spray and arrange on a baking sheet.

Melt the butter and chocolate in a heavy saucepan over medium-low heat; gently whisk until smooth. Remove from the heat and set aside.

Beat the eggs, egg yolk, vanilla, Splenda, and salt using a handheld mixer set at the highest speed until the volume is nearly tripled and the mixture has the texture of softly whipped cream, 7 to 8 minutes. Sprinkle the flour over the egg mixture and beat until just blended in. Pour the melted chocolate and butter into the egg mixture and gently fold until well blended and fairly uniform in color.

Spoon the batter into the prepared ramekins. Bake for 9 to 10 minutes, until the sides of the cakes have puffed slightly above the top edge of the ramekins but the centers are still soft. Do not overbake. Let the cakes cool for 1 minute, then unmold onto a dessert plate. Serve at once. A cooled cake is the texture of a very good fudge brownie and is delicious as well.

cooking for the holidays

Our fondest memories often center around holidays. We all have family traditions that make our celebrations special, and food is typically the basis of these customs. Most of us fear that our family holiday celebrations are over once we have had our bariatric weight-loss surgery. This is not true! The biggest change at my Christmas dinner table was that I was wearing clothes that were nine sizes smaller than the previous Christmas. It can be challenging, but with some planning and adjustments, we can prepare a fabulous holiday meal that we can enjoy every bit as much as the rest of our family and friends.

I was just six months post-op when my first holiday season rolled around. My Thanksgiving celebration was a disaster because I didn't have control over the kitchen. The foods that my in-laws prepared were all wrong for me and I couldn't eat many of the dishes—they either had too much sugar or were too dry. When I returned home I was determined to come up with delicious holiday recipes so that my Christmas celebration the next month would be spectacular. Here are suggestions for Thanksgiving, Christmas, and other holiday dinners and parties, prepared with love to celebrate the spirit of new health and happiness!

Holiday eating can be a problem for most of us. Pay attention to carbohydrates and watch for hidden sugar. I swore post-op that I would never prepare special diet meals just for myself. The changes that I have made to the menu to meet my needs are healthier for everyone at the table. So once again I am not the loner eating the soup!

Thanksgiving Menu

Thanksgiving is the most difficult holiday to reconstruct, as families have deeply ingrained food traditions and don't like anyone fooling around with their mama's Pink Salad recipe. I have found that the best way to handle the feast is to make sure that among all the heavy carbohydrate dishes, there is some moist turkey, flavorful gravy, sugar-free cranberry sauce, and sugar-free pumpkin pie that I can eat. You can't eat much but you can enjoy it a lot.

roasted turkey

5-ounce portion dark meat: Calories 260, fat 10 gr, carbs 0 gr, protein 40 gr
5-ounce portion white meat: Calories 219, fat 4 gr, carbs 0 gr, protein 42 gr
Serves 8 with leftovers

For a post-op person to enjoy this meal, it is imperative to have a perfectly roasted turkey. Just about everyone I know overcooks their turkey. An instant-read meat thermometer is key. Roast your turkey until a thigh reads 170°F and you will be astonished by the moistness of your bird. Even before my bariatric surgery, I would take a meat thermometer as a hostess gift when invited as a holiday dinner guest. Brining poultry guarantees moist and tender meat; a kosher turkey has already basically been brined in the koshering and salting process, and is very moist and juicy.

2 tablespoons salted butter

2 teaspoons Bell's Seasoning

One 12- to 15-pound kosher turkey, with neck and wing tips reserved
    for gravy, rinsed and thoroughly dried (Empire is a good brand)

Kosher salt and freshly ground black pepper

Preheat the oven to 425°F. Melt the butter in a small saucepan and
stir in the Bell's Seasoning. Place the turkey on a rack in a large roasting pan; dry the skin with paper towels, brush with the seasoned
butter, and lightly season with salt and pepper. Roast for 1 hour;
reduce the oven temperature to 325°F and continue to roast until an
instant-read thermometer inserted into the thickest part of the thigh
registers 170°F, 2½ to 3 hours. Remove the pan from the oven; carefully transfer the turkey to a platter, lightly covered with foil, and set
aside for 20 to 30 minutes to allow the juices to be reabsorbed into
the meat before carving.

pan gravy I

Per ¼-cup serving: Calories 47, fat 3 gr, carbs 3 gr, protein 1 gr
Makes approximately 2 cups

I always thought gravy was pretty important before having
my gastric surgery, but now it is essential if I am even going to
attempt to eat turkey. It is easy to make excellent gravy.

Turkey neck and wing tips, removed from the turkey after
    washing and drying

2 celery stalks

2 carrots

1 large onion, quartered

1 bay leaf

Several sprigs fresh thyme
12 whole peppercorns
2 cups chicken broth (see Note, page 127)
Pan drippings from roasted turkey
2 tablespoons cornstarch mixed with 3 tablespoons cold water
Kosher salt and freshly ground black pepper

Place the turkey neck and wing tips, celery, carrots, onion, bay leaf, thyme, peppercorns, and chicken broth in a medium saucepan, add 3 cups water, and bring to a boil over medium-high heat. Skim any foam that rises to the surface, lower the heat, and simmer for 60 to 90 minutes while the turkey is roasting, until the volume is reduced by half and the stock is flavorful. Strain through a fine-mesh sieve, pressing down on the solids to extract as much liquid as possible.

Once the turkey is done and transferred to the platter, spoon out and discard as much fat from the roasting pan as you can, and strain the pan drippings into the turkey stock. Bring the stock and drippings to a boil and whisk in enough of the cornstarch mixture to bring the gravy to your desired consistency. Season with salt and pepper.

pan gravy II

Per ¼-cup serving: Calories 29, fat 0.5 gr, carbs 5 gr,
protein <1 gr
Makes approximately 2 cups

When I roast a turkey breast and don't have the extra parts to make stock, I improvise and doctor up a packaged gravy.

1 tablespoon salted butter
½ pound cremini mushrooms, sliced
1 package Knorr Roasted Turkey gravy mix

2 tablespoons dry sherry

½ teaspoon garlic powder

Kosher salt and freshly ground black pepper

Pan drippings from roasted turkey or turkey breast, optional

Heat the butter in a medium nonstick skillet over medium-high heat until foaming. Add the mushrooms and sauté until the released liquid has evaporated and the mushrooms start to brown. Prepare the Knorr gravy mix in a medium saucepan according to the package directions. Add the sautéed mushrooms, sherry, and garlic powder. Simmer for 2 to 3 minutes, until the gravy is bubbling hot. Add ½ cup of defatted pan drippings, if desired, to punch up the flavor.

southern-style green beans

Per ½-cup serving: Calories 21, fat 0 gr, carbs 5 gr, protein 1 gr
Makes eight ½-cup servings

Green beans are low-carb, and when simmered the way my husband's Georgia family does it, albeit without fatback or lard, they are tender and incredibly delicious. The smoked turkey adds great flavor; most supermarkets now carry this product. I mash a few beans with my finely cut shreds of turkey for a moist mouthful. I don't make green beans any other way!

1 small onion, diced

1 teaspoon olive oil

¼-pound piece smoked turkey, cut from a wing or drumstick

1 teaspoon Cajun or Creole seasoning page 165

2 pounds fresh green beans, cut into 1-inch pieces

Kosher salt and freshly ground black pepper

Sauté the onion in the olive oil in a saucepan over medium heat until soft. Add the smoked turkey, Cajun seasoning, and green beans; cover with water. Bring the beans to a boil, set the lid on the pan slightly ajar, lower the heat, and simmer for 40 minutes, or until the liquid is almost evaporated and the beans are very tender. Season with salt and pepper.

roasted sweet potatoes

WLS portion (¼ small potato): Calories 40, fat 0 gr, carbs 10 gr, protein 1 gr
Serves 8

If you are going to eat carbs, make them count with good nutrition and lots of vitamins and minerals. I love sweet potatoes, and the silky, smooth texture satisfies my urge for potato. These salt-crusted roasted potatoes stay very hot while the turkey rests and you do your last-minute dinner preparations. To serve, cut a lengthwise slit in the potato and push the pointed ends toward the center, creating a pool for the butter and syrup for your dinner guests. I gild mine with a pat of butter and a drizzle of Steel's Sugar-Free Country Syrup (see Note)—two bites of heaven. No one in your family will miss the pecan, brown sugar, and marshmallow topping, and they will all be healthier for skipping it.

8 small sweet potatoes
Olive oil
Kosher salt

Preheat the oven to 400°F. Rub each sweet potato with a little olive oil, sprinkle with salt, and place on a baking sheet. Roast for 40 to 60 minutes, until the potatoes feel soft when the sides are pressed.

Note: Steel's Gourmet Foods produces a line of sugar-free cooking sauces, sweeteners, and exceptional syrups that do not raise blood sugar levels and are excellent products for anyone who limits sugar intake. The most important feature of these sauces and syrups is the taste; the ingredients read like recipes rather than lists of chemicals and additives. These are sugar-free products that are truly worth eating! (For information, see Sources, page 303.)

cranberry sauce

Per 2-tablespoon serving: Calories 10, fat 0 gr, carbs 4.5 gr, protein <1 gr
Makes approximately 2 cups

Make this a day or two ahead. No need for canned sauce when this sugar-free version is so quick and tasty. My husband prefers a smooth cranberry sauce, so I puree the sauce and pour it into a straight-sided glass to chill. To serve, I dip the glass into hot water for 20 seconds, cover with a dish, flip to unmold, and slice.

2 teaspoons unflavored gelatin (about ⅔ packet)
Juice and rinds of 1 orange (about ⅓ cup juice)
One 12-ounce package fresh cranberries
1 cup Splenda Granular

Sprinkle the gelatin over 2 tablespoons water in a small measuring cup and set aside for 2 minutes without stirring. Quarter the orange rinds. Combine the cranberries, orange juice, orange rinds, and ½ cup water in a medium saucepan, and cook over medium-high heat for about 10 minutes, until the berries pop and the mixture is very soft. Remove from the heat, remove and discard the orange rinds, and stir in the Splenda and the gelatin mixture until dissolved. Transfer to a decorative bowl or mold and chill for several hours or overnight.

pumpkin pie

Full portion: Calories 113, fat 5 gr, carbs 12 gr, protein 3.5 gr
Makes 2 pies, each serving 8

Here's the famous Libby's label-on-the-can version with some adjustments. Sugar acts as a preservative in desserts; because this pie is sugar-free it *must* be kept in the refrigerator. This pie tastes like Thanksgiving and works for even the most recent post-op people.

2 cups sugar-free gingersnap cookies (Murray is a widely available supermarket brand)
2 tablespoons salted butter, melted
Spiced Pumpkin Custard (page 265)
Whipped cream sweetened with Splenda

Preheat the oven to 325°F. Place the cookies in a food processor and pulse with the butter until you have moist, fine crumbs. Divide the mixture and press evenly into two 8-inch pie plates. Bake for 10 to 12 minutes, until the crusts just start to color. Cool on a rack while preparing the filling. Leave the oven on at 325°F.

Divide the pumpkin custard filling between the two pie plates. Bake for 20 to 25 minutes, until the filling is set around the edges and the center is still a bit soft. Transfer to a rack to cool, then chill. Serve with a dollop of Splenda-sweetened whipped cream.

amazing pecan pie

Full portion: Calories 171, fat 14.5 gr, carbs 7.5 gr, protein 3 gr
Serves 10

The amazing thing about this pie is that it's sugar-free! The
ingredient list is specific, and substitutions won't work. To
make this pie you need Steel's Sugar-Free Country Maple Syrup,
which can be ordered online (see Sources, page 303). When I
tried to make this recipe using other brands of sugar-free syrup,
the custard became muddy and, quite frankly, tasted awful. The
Steel's syrup is very thick, and that makes a huge difference.
Even though this pie is sweet, it doesn't have any sugar to act as a
preservative, so it must be kept in the refrigerator, or it will spoil
quickly.

3 large eggs
¾ cup Splenda Granular
Pinch of table salt
1 teaspoon vanilla extract
4 tablespoons salted butter, melted
¾ cup Steel's Sugar-Free Country Maple Syrup
½ cup chopped pecans, plus 10 halves
One 9-inch homemade unbaked pie shell, or store bought frozen
      prepared (I use Mrs. Smith's)
Whipped cream sweetened with Splenda

Preheat the oven to 350°F. Beat the eggs in a large bowl until well
blended and stir in the Splenda, salt, vanilla, butter, and syrup. Mix
in the chopped pecans and pour the filling into the pie crust. Arrange
the pecan halves evenly on the custard and bake for 30 to 35 minutes,

until the sides are set but the center is still a bit soft. Cool to room temperature and serve in small wedges with Splenda-sweetened whipped cream.

Christmas and Holiday Party Menu

I have put together this party menu, keeping in mind our food requirements. We can eat all of these foods but, more important, our guests will enjoy them as well. Every single item is moist, easy to eat, and low in carbohydrates, making it a good food choice for someone who has had weight-loss surgery.

cocktail hour
Teriyaki Cheese Log with sesame flatbread crackers and
     crudités
Spiced Roasted Pecans
Ultimate Bloody Marys

dinner
Shrimp Louis Cocktail
Garlic-Herb Beef Tenderloin with Roasted Garlic Cream
Roasted Asparagus
Crisp Green Onion and Parmesan Polenta Cakes

dessert table
Individual Almond-Crusted Cheesecakes with Black Cherry
     Compote
Eggnog
Coffee with DaVinci sugar-free syrups

teriyaki cheese log

WLS portion (1 tablespoon): Calories 50, fat 4 gr, carbs 2 gr, protein 2 gr
Makes about 1 cup

This simple and delicious cheese dip is excellent party food. Surround the log with sesame flatbread crackers and cucumber slices and garnish with green-onion brushes.

½ pound reduced-fat cream cheese, at room temperature
1 tablespoon grated peeled fresh ginger
3 green onions (scallions), minced
½ teaspoon garlic powder
1 tablespoon soy sauce
Sesame seeds

In a large bowl, beat together the cream cheese, ginger, green onions, garlic powder, and soy sauce until thoroughly combined. Chill until firm, 30 to 40 minutes. Transfer the mixture to a piece of wax paper and roll into a log shape. Spread the sesame seeds in a shallow dish, then place the cheese log on the seeds and roll to coat. Wrap and chill until ready to serve.

spiced roasted pecans

Per serving, 6 to 8 nuts: Calories 54, fat 2.5 gr, carbs 1 gr,
protein <1 gr
Makes 2 cups

These toasted nuts are addictive. Since Ty's family lives in the
heart of a prime pecan-growing region, I always keep a supply on
hand in my freezer. I make this recipe in large batches and pack
them in decorative tins for holiday gifts or hostess gifts.

2 tablespoons salted butter
1 teaspoon Worcestershire sauce
½ teaspoon garlic powder
½ teaspoon Tabasco sauce
2 tablespoons Steel's Sugar-Free Country Maple Syrup,
    or 2 tablespoons Splenda Granular
2 cups unbroken pecan halves
Kosher salt

Preheat the oven to 300°F. Melt the butter in a small saucepan and
stir in the Worcestershire, garlic powder, Tabasco, and syrup. Pour
over the pecans in a medium bowl and toss to evenly coat. Spread the
nuts in a single layer on a baking sheet, generously sprinkle with salt,
and bake, stirring occasionally, until the nuts are crisp and toasted,
20 to 25 minutes. Cool the pecans on the baking sheet, breaking up
any that stick together. Store in an airtight container.

ultimate bloody marys

Full portion: Calories 80, fat 0 gr, carbs 4 gr, protein<1 gr
Makes enough spice paste for 20 cocktails

I often serve these tasty Bloody Marys when we have guests for dinner, and I have included them in my Holiday Party Menu as a cocktail-hour drink. They contain no sugar and no carbonation, and they still taste great with a half portion of pepper-flavored vodka. Skip the vodka altogether, and you have a deliciously spiced Virgin Bloody Mary.

This recipe works well for a party. Prepare a bowl of the highly spiced seasoning and let your guests flavor their cocktails as mildly or boldly as they like.

1 cup grated prepared horseradish

2 tablespoons A.1. steak sauce

2 tablespoons Worcestershire sauce

1½ tablespoons Tabasco sauce

1 tablespoon celery salt

1½ teaspoons coarsely ground black pepper

1 tablespoon fresh lemon juice

1 tablespoon chipotle chile powder, or 1 tablespoon Tabasco
　　Chipotle hot sauce

Absolut Peppar vodka

Tomato juice

Lemon slices

Green olives

Blend the horseradish, A.1., Worcestershire, Tabasco, celery salt, pepper, lemon juice, and chipotle powder in a medium bowl until smooth. Combine 1 tablespoon of the spice paste with 1 ounce of Absolut Peppar vodka and blend with 8 ounces of tomato juice. Pour the mixture over ice in a tall glass and garnish with lemon slices and olives.

shrimp louis cocktail

WLS ½ portion: Calories 75, fat 5 gr, carbs 3 gr, protein 10 gr
Serves 8

Be gentle when you coat the shrimp mixture with the sauce; the avocado cubes will mash if you are too aggressive. Use a large silicone spatula to carefully fold in the ingredients.

½ cup light mayonnaise
¼ cup bottled chili sauce
1 garlic clove, mashed with a pinch of salt
1 tablespoon fresh lime juice
1 teaspoon Tabasco sauce
Kosher salt and freshly ground black pepper
1½ pounds large shrimp, lightly poached, peeled, and deveined
1 medium Hass avocado, peeled and cut into ½-inch cubes
2 tablespoons minced red onion
2 cups watercress, trimmed, washed, and thoroughly dried
2 green onions (scallions), thinly sliced
2 hard-cooked eggs, quartered
Lime slices

In a large bowl, whisk together the mayonnaise, chili sauce, garlic, lime juice, and Tabasco until smooth; season with salt and pepper. Gently toss the shrimp, avocado, and red onion with about two-thirds of the sauce. Place a small bed of watercress in each of 8 large martini glasses or serving plates, and place a scoop of the shrimp mixture on top. Drizzle with some of the remaining sauce, sprinkle with the green onion slices, and garnish with a wedge of egg and a slice of lime.

garlic-herb beef tenderloin with roasted garlic cream

Per 3½ ounce portion: Calories 200, fat 12 gr, carbs 1 gr, protein 22 gr
Serves 8 to 10

Beef tenderloin is a perfect entrée for a party or special occasion; it is simple to season, effortless to roast to the perfect degree of doneness, and uncomplicated to carve. This main course is ready in under an hour, so make sure your side dishes are under control before placing the beef in the oven.

2 whole garlic bulbs
1 whole fillet of beef (tenderloin), 3½ to 4 pounds
3 garlic cloves
2 tablespoons fresh rosemary, leaves only
2 tablespoons fresh thyme, leaves only
2 medium shallots
Kosher salt and freshly ground black pepper
2 tablespoons olive oil
1 cup reduced-fat sour cream

Preheat the oven to 400°F. Wrap the 2 whole garlic bulbs in foil and roast until soft, 45 to 60 minutes. Remove from the oven, unwrap, and set aside to cool.

Trim the tenderloin of excess fat and any tough outer silver skin. Tuck the thinner, tapered tip under the roast and firmly tie the entire tenderloin with cotton butcher's string at 2-inch intervals.

Turn the oven up to 425°F. Make an herb paste by combining the raw garlic cloves, rosemary, thyme, shallots, 1½ teaspoons salt, 2 teaspoons coarsely ground black pepper, and the olive oil in a food processor. Place the tenderloin in a heavy roasting pan and evenly coat the roast with the herb paste. Roast to an internal temperature of 120°F for perfect medium-rare doneness, 30 to 35 minutes. Remove the tenderloin from the oven and allow the meat to rest for at least 15 minutes (longer is fine) before carving into slices.

When the roasted garlic is cool enough to handle, squeeze the garlic from each clove into a small bowl and stir to make a smooth puree. Blend in the sour cream and season with salt and plenty of black pepper. Serve the herbed beef tenderloin at room temperature with the sauce.

roasted asparagus

Per 4-spear portion: Calories 15, fat 2 gr, carbs 3 gr, protein 1 gr
Serves 8

Roasting asparagus intensifies its flavor and makes the spears easy to eat.

2 pounds fresh asparagus, bottoms trimmed and peeled
1 tablespoon olive oil
1 teaspoon balsamic vinegar
Kosher salt and freshly ground black pepper

Preheat the oven to 500°F. Toss the asparagus with the olive oil and vinegar in a large bowl, and place them in a single layer on a baking

sheet. Season with salt and pepper. Roast for 12 minutes, or until
the asparagus are tender when pierced with the tip of a knife, but still
firm. Transfer to a serving platter.

crisp green onion
and parmesan polenta cakes

WLS ½ portion: Calories 60, fat 3.5 gr, carbs 7.5 gr, protein 1 gr
Makes 9 polenta squares

A perfect counterpart to the roasted tenderloin for the folks not
watching their carbohydrates. Now that I am several years post-
surgery, I will have a small portion of this delicious dish. If I am
going to have a carbohydrate, I want to be sure it is delectable.
Who wants to waste their precious few carbohydrate grams on
boring mashed potatoes? This dish can be prepared in advance
to the point of refrigerating the seasoned polenta mixture; leave
the cutting and browning of the cakes for last-minute preparation
while the asparagus spears roast.

2 tablespoons salted butter
1 cup stone-ground polenta or yellow stone-ground grits
    (see Note, page 168)
2 bunches green onions (scallions), thinly sliced
2 tablespoons olive oil
½ cup freshly grated Parmesan
Kosher salt and freshly ground black pepper
Vegetable oil cooking spray
All-purpose or Wondra flour for dusting

Lightly spray a 9-inch square baking pan with cooking spray.

Bring 5 cups of water and the butter to a boil in a large saucepan over medium-high heat. Slowly whisk in the polenta, stirring constantly to prevent lumping. Reduce the heat to low, cover, and simmer, stirring frequently, until the polenta is tender, about 30 minutes.

While the polenta is cooking, sauté the green onions in 1 tablespoon of the olive oil in a medium saucepan until soft, about 4 minutes. Set aside.

Remove the polenta from the heat, stir in the green onions and Parmesan, and season with salt and pepper. Pour into the prepared baking pan, smooth the top, and refrigerate until firm, about 2 hours. Turn the firm polenta out onto a piece of plastic wrap, and cut into 9 squares.

Heat the remaining tablespoon of olive oil in a large nonstick skillet over medium-high heat. Lightly dust the top and bottom of each polenta square with flour, add to the pan in a single layer, and cook until brown and crisp, about 4 minutes per side.

individual almond-crusted cheesecakes with black cherry compote

Full portion: Calories 196, fat 14 gr, carbs 10 gr, protein 7 gr
Serves 10

A fabulous pairing of almond and cherry shines in the perfect ending for this holiday feast. It is so simple to make these individual cakes in advance and keep them on a tray in the refrigerator until dessert time. No complicated serving preparations or cutting—just unmold and pour on a little of the cherry sauce.

Vegetable oil cooking spray

1½ cups Joseph's Sugar-Free Almond cookies (see Note, page 241)

1 tablespoon salted butter, softened, at room temparature

1½ pounds reduced-fat cream cheese, at room temperature

1¾ cups Splenda Granular

1 teaspoon almond extract

2 teaspoons vanilla extract

½ cup reduced-fat sour cream

3 large eggs plus 1 additional yolk, lightly beaten

½ cup sliced almonds

2 cups pitted fresh black cherries, sliced (or frozen, unthawed)

2 teaspoons cornstarch

2 tablespoons amaretto

Preheat the oven to 325°F. Lightly spray ten 6-ounce heavy foil baking cups with cooking spray.

In a food processor, grind the almond cookies until they are the texture of fine bread crumbs. Blend in the butter. Press a couple of tablespoons of the crust crumbs into each of the prepared foil cups. Place on a baking sheet and bake for 6 to 8 minutes, until the crusts just start to color.

Using an electric mixer, beat the cream cheese until smooth; add 1½ cups of the Splenda, the almond extract, vanilla, sour cream, and eggs, beating thoroughly after each addition. Scrape down the bowl and blend again until smooth. Fill each cup two-thirds full, place a few sliced almonds on each cake, and bake for 18 to 20 minutes, or until the center is barely set. Place the baking sheet on a rack and cool to room temperature. Chill in the refrigerator for at least 2 hours before serving.

Bring the cherries, the remaining ¼ cup of Splenda, and ¼ cup water to a boil in a medium saucepan; lower the heat and simmer. Blend the cornstarch with the amaretto in a small cup and add to the cherry mixture, stirring constantly until the mixture thickens and becomes glossy. Transfer to a small bowl and chill before using.

Unmold each cheesecake onto a dessert plate, and spoon on some of the cherry sauce.

eggnog

Full portion: Calories 80, fat 2 gr, carbs 6 gr, protein 4.5 gr
Makes twelve ½-cup servings

6 cups 2% low-fat milk
1 cup Splenda Granular
6 egg yolks
1 tablespoon vanilla extract
Freshly grated nutmeg
¼ cup dark rum or amaretto

Whisk together 5 cups of the milk and ½ cup of the Splenda in a medium saucepan and bring the mixture just to the simmering point over medium heat. Beat the egg yolks with the remaining ½ cup of Splenda in a medium bowl and, whisking constantly, slowly pour in half of the hot milk, blending until smooth. Pour the eggs and milk back into the saucepan, whisking until well combined. Place the saucepan over medium-low heat and, stirring constantly, cook until the custard is thick enough to coat the back of a spoon, 6 to

8 minutes; it should never boil. Remove from the heat and stir in the vanilla and ½ teaspoon freshly grated nutmeg. Cool slightly. Pour the mixture though a fine-mesh strainer into a bowl or pitcher, cover, and chill. Just before serving, stir in the rum and the additional 1 cup milk, if necessary, to achieve the desired consistency. Serve in small glasses with a generous grating of nutmeg.

sources

When you first get involved in the process of having weight-loss surgery, it is overwhelming to wade through all of the information to figure out what you need in the way of protein drinks, vitamins, and mineral supplements. It is common to be dazed and confused by the volume of products on the market. There are protein powders and bars that are wrong for our needs, and then there are those that are appropriate by the numbers but taste terrible; we don't all need to repeat the same mistakes and waste money by buying them.

This is why I have created a companion website to this book where we've brought together the newest and best products that we need in order to be successful in our bariatric journey. I use protein supplements every day, I take daily vitamins, and I use sugar-free products to prepare meals for my family. We only carry products that combine good taste with great nutrition, and every single item on my website is one that I have personally selected and evaluated for appropriateness along with the results from my team of bariatric post-op taste testers.

It is the best resource not only for excellent-tasting protein drinks, the right vitamin supplements, and sugar-free foods that are worth eating, but also for recipes, support, and information that affects our health. The top bariatric practices recommend **BariatricEating.com** to their patients, and we are proud to be a Corporate Council member of the American Society for Bariatric Surgery (ASBS) and closely follow the latest medical findings that impact our pre- and post-surgical lives.

In response to the tremendous need for positive support and accurate information, we have launched a message board that is accessible from our BariatricEating.com website and also can be located directly at **BeforeAndAfterHelp.com.**

The message board is for you! Many successful post-ops are there to answer your questions, calm your fears, explain the little aches and pains, motivate you to walk a mile, share the latest protein latte recipe, suggest a soft food for day 14, give you a gentle hug, lead the applause for celebrating success—or give you a swift kick in the pants if you are out of control.

You'll find thousands of bariatric patients assembled in a forum offering encouragement to those struggling with post-operative lifestyle changes. With increased focus on aftercare, we find that many just need the assurance of someone who not only has talked the talk, but has walked the walk. If you have enjoyed this book, you will love both our website and message board!

Nutritional Analysis

A superb source of nutrition and fitness information is located online at **FitDay.com.** It is an excellent place for you to keep a daily record of the foods you eat and the exercise you get. Based on your journal entries, this website analyzes your diet, exercise, and weight loss and generates easy-to-read charts and tables tracking your short- and long-term progress. I love the "Today's Foods" section; I can add up every morsel I put into my mouth and get a total nutritional breakdown. There is no ignoring too many carbs or too little protein with this feature.

Protein-Rich Products

protein powders

Experiment with protein powders to find one that you like before you have your surgery. Do not choose a protein supplement that is high in carbohydrates; these formulations are for bodybuilders, not people with bariatric weight loss. Low carbohydrate content is crucial for us, so read the label and choose a powder that contains no more than 7 to 9 grams of carbs per shake and delivers at least 20 grams of protein per scoop. Please also remember that you get what you pay for with protein—the cheap bags and kegs of protein shake mix are not high quality and your body will not benefit from what you believe you are consuming.

Do not bother with the liquid gelatin-type plastic tubes of protein. While it was once thought that these collagen bullets were a great concentrated source of protein, we now know that *collagen protein* does not contain the complete range of amino acids that can be either absorbed or used by the body. As the price of top-quality whey protein isolate increased over the years, manufacturers scrambled to find a cheap and readily available form of protein, and this product came into use. Collagen protein is made from rendered animal hides and joints. Manufacturers attempt to hide the protein source and often disguise the collagen content by using words such as *isolated collagen* to confuse consumers, or they even list a protein blend in the ingredients that contains a tiny amount of whey protein isolate so they can boast that their product contains isolate on the front label when in fact it is nearly all collagen. If a manufacturer is not clear or tries to hide or invent a new name for the protein source, there is a problem.

I developed my own line of protein drinks because I use protein drinks when I go to the gym and when I travel, and I only want the purest and best tasting for my own needs. Inspire whey protein isolate drink mixes and Pure Unflavored Whey Protein Isolate are made with clean, pure whey protein isolate. Whey protein isolate is the most bioavailable form of protein. This means that what you drink is going to be absorbed into your body and not wasted—it is extremely efficient.

You can check our website for stores where Inspire whey protein isolate drink mixes, soup mixes, and Pure Unflavored Whey Protein Isolate powder are sold, but they are always available on **www.BeHealthyDrinks.com**.

Inspire Pure Whey Protein Isolate Drink Flavors
Peanut Butter Cookie
Dutch Chocolate Cake
Chocolate Peanut Butter Fudge
Cinnamon Cappuccino
Caramel Latte
Hot Chocolate with Marshmallows
Apple Pie
Ice Cream Sandwich
Vanilla Date
Pomegranate Berry
Tangerine Pineapple
Raspberry Lemonade
Strawberry Lemonade
Summer Melon
Pistachio
Natural Vanilla Very Berry
Natural Northern Lights Espresso
Natural Vanilla Cookie

Inspire Soups Fortified with Pure Whey Protein Isolate
Mexican Taco
Lasagna

Asian Chicken
Tomato Bisque

ready-to-drink protein

Grab-and-go protein drinks are a true convenience in our busy world. While they are more expensive, there is nothing like popping the top of a can or bottle and having a smooth, delicious protein drink.

Believe ready-to-drink bottled lattes, vanilla, and chai tea are a delicious premium blend with 20 grams of protein, just a few grams of carbs depending on the flavor, and zero fat. These delicious Splenda-sweetened protein latte drinks contain 500 mg of calcium and a big hit of natural energy from B vitamins, and are virtually indistinguishable from a bottled Starbucks Frappuccino. Believe has Italian Cappuccino, Mocha Latte, Smooth Chai Tea, and Vanilla Creme Brulee flavors—and Mango, Chocolate, and Coconut are in the works.

Availability of RTDs is ever changing, so we recommend your checking our website for the latest products that taste great and fit our post-operative needs.

protein bars

Used sparingly as portable protein, protein bars are a much better choice than fast food or sugary snacks. They're a good nutritional tool as long as they're a planned part of your diet, not a mindless snack. I keep bars in my purse and in my car, and I make sure that I have one for the mall or several in my bag for airline travel, as I've been stuck in a small foreign airport for hours with zero food options.

Do not eat protein bars that are high in sugar and carbs. There are many formulations that are intentionally high in carbs for body-builders and athletes; these are *not* the ones you want. I see bariatric patients nibbling on Balance and Luna bars with 20 to 40 grams of sugar, and it just makes me shake my head. The low-sugar bars are usually in their own section, have fewer than 10 net or impact carbs and 12 to 30 grams of protein, and some actually taste good!

There have been great improvements in the many years I've been using protein bars. I used to look for the bar that was the least objectionable, and the choice was between peanut butter- or chocolate-flavored clay. Today there are bars available that taste like candy bars. Beware that the sugar alcohols in many bars—glycerine, maltitol, glycerol—can have an explosive gas or laxative effect on many people.

There's always great change in the availability of new protein or nutrition bars, so it's best that you check our website for the latest protein bars that not only taste good but contain the proper nutrition for our surgery. I rely on Power Crunch, Quest, Supreme, and, in a pinch at an airport or hotel lobby shop, Luna LemonZest bars.

Vitamins and Minerals

We have to take good-quality vitamin supplements for the rest of our lives because of our potential for deficiencies. Statistics are alarming, with a recent study showing that 98 percent of gastric bypass post-ops having two or more deficiencies after the second year.

Through my many years in dealing with bariatric patients, it came to my attention that all too many of us say we take our supplements when we don't. The companies that manufacture bariatric-specific supplements keep adding on more bottles of supplements for us to take rather than reformulating to include the nutrient that is lacking. Understandable from a corporate view, but difficult from a patient view for practical purposes.

At times I kept as many as nine individual bottles of supplements on my desk and rarely took them. I could not deal with big chalky calcium tablets and hated the strong kids' sour fruit taste of the rest of the lot. I knew I needed to take them but found it impossible to follow the recommended schedule for what supplements interacted with the others and how many hours apart some tablets needed to be chewed. It made me feel like a failure—and because so many of us cover up our shortcomings, the guilt and shame rolled in.

With my background in blood chemistry, I knew there had to be mineral forms that worked for when and how we needed to take our nutrients. I wanted my formulations to contain the highest-quality form of each ingredient, not the cheapest obtainable sourced from China.

I began working with the specialists at Albion minerals in Utah and discovered that their highly absorbable, organic forms of critical trace minerals and patented chelates were used by hematologists and medical specialists in dealing with severe cases of anemia and deficiencies throughout the world.

When choosing your daily nutrition, pay attention to whether the company is simply trying to make money or if it was started by someone who had a health problem helped by nutrition. People who have started companies to help others get healthy usually make great vitamins, as they know firsthand what quality nutrients can do and benefit from using their own products! I was motivated to create Journey when I was at a surgeon's conference and I asked a top vitamin executive why he didn't use specialized chelated minerals that appeared to be a solution to our deficiencies, and he plainly replied, "Cost." At that moment I knew I had to be my own advocate.

All these years, I've been thinking about the day when I would be in a position to work with supplement experts to create a product line that:

- Was easy to take
- Used fewer tablets or capsules
- Included forms of minerals that didn't interact
- Was efficient, so that smaller volumes could be used
- Could be made into smaller, less obnoxious-size tablets with better textures

I am proud of the Journey Bariatric and Journey Essentials lines of supplements and that they have solved the supplement problem for so many of us. For the first time I take my supplements every day, and my health, including my hair and nails, is so much better as a result. Our health needs to be in the hands of the best nutrition we can find.

Journey Bariatric Multiformula Berry Melts
Journey Bariatric Multiformula Capsules
Journey Essentials Calcium and D Lemon Melts
Journey Essentials Dimacal® Calcium and D Capsules
Journey Essentials Gentle Iron Grape Melts
Journey Essentials Gentle Iron Capsules
Journey Essentials Tummy Balance Strawberry Melts
Journey Essentials Vitamin D$_3$ Essence Drops
Journey Essentials Hair Balance Capsules
Journey Essentials Sleep Balance Natural Rest Enhancer Lemon
  Lime Melts

Plastic Surgery

It seems like yesterday when I was sitting in the plastic surgeon's waiting room while my girlfriend JoAnne underwent the second of her three planned reconstructive procedures: a lower body lift, medial and lateral thigh life, and upper arm lift.

At noon, we entered the pre-surgical suite, and within a few minutes, the anesthesiologist (not a nurse anesthetist, but an M.D.) started her IV. Then Jo, a beautiful sixty-eight-year-old who was in love with her new slimmer and much healthier life, gave me a hug and shuffled into the operating room. She was then in the strong and capable hands of a top plastic surgeon in the specialty of post-gastric bypass reconstruction. Surgeons like Dr. Bernard Shuster understand skin challenges that remain after a loss of 100 pounds or more and have perfected techniques to not only safely remove excess skin but also leave a pleasing result. These are technically difficult procedures often requiring extensive reconstruction, as the surgeons are not starting with a smooth or blank canvas. Dr. Shuster is one of a select group of surgeons playing an integral role in our recovery by providing not just ordinary but outstanding surgical results for postoperative bariatric patients.

I remember an old message board thread started by a gastric bypass post-op who had gone for a plastic surgery consult. She was upset that the doctor told her that she wouldn't have a belly button after her tummy tuck procedure, as he didn't "do" belly buttons. This bothered her and she asked for opinions and support. She actually felt silly and ungrateful for wanting to have a belly button after her tummy tuck! As I read the first fifteen or so responses, I could feel my eyebrows begin to rise and fingers itch for my keyboard, as there was not one post that encouraged her to find another surgeon for another opinion. All the replies to her post encouraged her to be happy that her insurance was going to cover her surgery and be satisfied that she was going to be rid of the large skin flap, and chided her for mourning the loss of her useless belly button.

I clenched my teeth as I contemplated the mind-set of these folks who didn't understand that they were the customer and that they got to approve or reject the planned result. They didn't realize that they should shop around and compare doctors' skills, attitudes, and areas of expertise. That even though this was plastic surgery, it was still an operation, and that they should expect at least reasonable results.

No belly button? This doesn't even make sense. How can a plastic surgeon worth their degree not be able to leave a patient with an intact belly button? More important, why wasn't anyone else upset about this? When you have a tummy tuck or abdominoplasty, your belly button isn't moved; the skin around it is. The surgeon first makes a horizontal incision between your belly button and pubic hairline, cuts around your belly button (known as your umbilicus), loosens the surrounding belly skin, pulls down the excess skin, and then cuts a hole in the skin so your belly button can once again peek through. So it is never detached—it stays put while the surrounding area is manipulated. Basically, an experienced plastic surgeon leaves you with a belly button—in fact, the same one you started out with. While I cannot say we are all left with an attractive belly button even with the best of plastic surgeons, at least we have one. (Perhaps a new technique needs to be discovered and shared so we don't end up with those odd bull's-eyes.)

We need to be educated consumers when it comes to medical procedures. We agonize over buying a vacuum cleaner or a blender, but don't investigate a gastric bypass surgeon or plastic surgeon because they happen to be listed in our insurance book. There are surgeons, good surgeons, and great surgeons; based on the numbers of procedures they perform, technique, schooling, innate capability, and results. Find a surgeon who is practiced in dealing with large amounts of excess skin. This is an art, and a surgeon who is gifted in this art, barring unforeseen circumstances, leaves you with a belly button. (Although there is a Victoria's Secret Angel who does not have a belly button, and it's said that one is Photoshopped in so that the photos do not look strange.) While I'm on a roll, I believe that a great plastic surgeon will not close your incision with staples. Plastic surgeons are proud of their delicate, nearly invisible perfect stitches. This is a hallmark of plastic surgery. Now this is just my opinion, but you would have to be out of your mind to allow a plastic surgeon to staple your abdominoplasty incision. Maybe (just maybe) if you were having extensive reconstructive procedures requiring several feet of incisions, this might justify staples. For the average tummy tuck, it is not acceptable, and I would leave the office of any surgeon who suggested it.

Did you know that any doctor who practices in any medical specialty can decide he is going to start doing brow lifts or even breast augmentations starting next Wednesday? Make sure your chosen surgeon is board certified in the specialty of plastic surgery and that he specializes in the procedure you're having done. Ask the surgeon directly how many tummy tucks, or thigh lifts, or body lifts he performs each month . . . each week. How many are on people who have lost 150 pounds? Do you really want someone who has never done an arm lift (called a brachioplasty) doing his first one on you? This is not a procedure to be taken lightly—I know a bariatric post-op who can't hold up her arms to drive without pain because of poor technique used by a surgeon who had never done a brachioplasty before. Her scars are thick ropes extending into her armpits, and they're not only visually disturbing, they compromise function.

Doing a tummy tuck on someone who has a little flab after having a baby is very different from reconstructing an 11-pound skin flap after a 219-pound weight loss. Don't choose a plastic surgeon who has never done a medial thigh lift—this is not a common procedure, and a poor outcome can affect your life. I know a patient who was very large below the waist and, after losing 230 pounds, was left with uncomfortable drooping skin folds on her inner and outer thighs. The small-town general surgeon she chose, who was not qualified to perform this difficult reconstructive procedure, left her with wide scars, gynecological complications, and the accompanying emotional distress. We've all heard that practice makes perfect, but studies prove it is true. Choose someone who is both qualified and practiced in the procedure you want or need.

Ask questions, don't be intimidated, and ask to see actual photos of the surgeon's patients so you can see how his procedures turn out. Some surgeons will actually give you the contact information of one or two of their patients who have had the procedure you are seeking. Please do not think for a moment that you should settle for what you can get because you're using an insurance benefit.

While your bariatric surgeon is often eager to recommend a plastic surgeon, they all too often recommend a colleague based on their relationship with them. When you're in your surgeon's support group, you can see live work on actual patients, so respectfully evaluate the results on people who share similar skin issues.

Stellar examples of plastic surgeons who specialize in bariatric patient skin removal are Dr. Bernard Shuster of Hollywood, Florida; Dr. Alan Pillersdorf of Palm Beach, Florida; and Dr. Timothy Katzen of Beverly Hills, California. I adore these men for their dedication to helping us! Maybe we should tell that Victoria's Secret Angel that all three of these fine surgeons do belly buttons!

A last thought . . . please, please, before you have that plastic surgery, *stop smoking,* take your vitamins, and consume plenty of protein so that your body can heal. Plan for your surgical success, and do everything you can to help your surgeon achieve the beautiful results you deserve.

- **www.DrShuster.net**—Make sure you check out his online secure photo consultation service. The doctor will speak with you personally. Dr. Shuster has turned out some of the best-looking post-brachioplasty arms I have seen—amazing results for a difficult procedure.
- **www.PlasticSurgeryPB.com**—Dr. Pillersdorf is a fine surgeon who is practiced in post-bariatric procedures.
- **www.BodyByKatzen.com**—I have known Dr. Katzen for many years; I know many of his satisfied and very happy patients. He has been featured on TLC's *The Real Skinny,* which followed several of his patients before and after multiple extreme reconstructive procedures following massive bariatric weight loss.

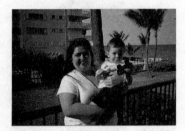

Before: 278 lbs.

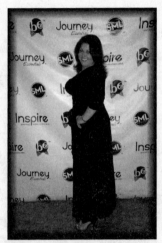

After: 147 lbs.

The eleven years since my surgery have flown by. I am still extremely mindful about my food choices but in a different direction. Rather than seeing how painfully low I can go with all carbs, I now strive for balance, eating simple clean unprocessed foods with lots of vegetables. It takes time to grasp the difference between Twinkie carbs and hummus carbs.

I am about thirty pounds more than my lowest weight—just when you have this figured out, along comes fifty and menopause changes the game and kicks your butt. That's life! Age is a privilege denied to many. I have eclipsed the age of my beautiful mother and am enjoying every minute of my journey.

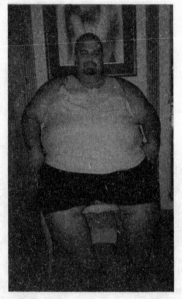 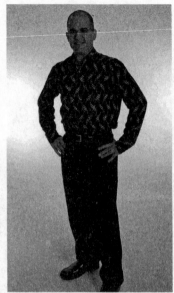

Before: 529 lbs.   After: 168 lbs.

I lost over 350 pounds! I started out with a body mass index of 77 and was classified as *super morbidly obese* at 529 pounds. Now I am 168 pounds and full of life. I went from a desk job at a local airline to being a flight attendant, not because it was my dream, but because at my highest weight I couldn't perform the duties of a flight attendant. Today my journey continues and I am an advocate for getting bariatric patients to understand that surgery is only half the battle. Nutrition, psychological health, and exercise play a crucial role in maintaining this new life.

Sarah Poppe

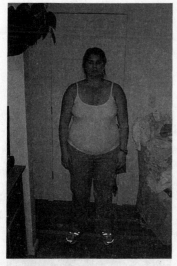 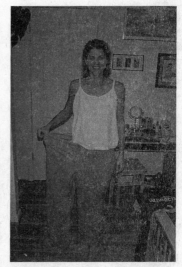

Before: 245 lbs.   After: 138 lbs.

Why didn't I just modify my eating and not have surgery? Why didn't I just exercise more before I had the surgery? Why did I take such a radical and risky path? I had open RNY gastric bypass surgery for my three children, my amazing husband, my mother, my sister, my nieces and nephew. I was in my early thirties and felt helpless and out of control for years, eating myself into oblivion. Today, I am in my forties and my re-birthday was November 17, 2005. My highest weight was 245 and my current weight is 138, which is perfect for my 5'7" frame. While shrinking on the outside, I am growing on the inside. Post-op life isn't easy. Now I taste the food, sample the texture, enjoy the smell. I have eaten better in the past year than ever before in my life. I also incorporated exercise into my life. I ran a 5-kilometer race! I always dreamed of running in a race, and now I have experienced crossing that finish line. Life is grand!

Julie Hedges

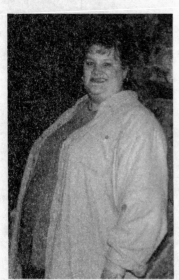

Before: 291 lbs.

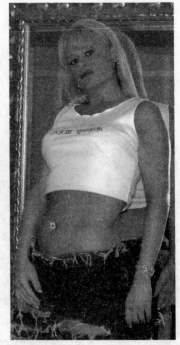

After: 147 lbs.

WLS has allowed me to become the active, successful, and confident individual that was hidden below layers of obesity. I have a successful business, a successful marriage, and soon a beautiful, healthy baby because I no longer allow myself to be burdened by the excuses that obesity allows. WLS was the best decision I ever made in my life. It provided me with a new freedom . . . releasing me from the stereotypes that other people have about obese people. I'm intelligent, independent, and sexy. What a blessing gastric bypass has been.

index